The DeFlame Diet
For Breast Health & Cancer Prevention

By David R. Seaman, DC, MS

Author of
The DeFlame Diet
&
Weight Loss Secrets You Need To Know

www.deflame.com

Shadow Panther Press

Wilmington, NC

Disclaimer

This book is intended as an educational volume only; not as a medical or treatment manual. The information contained herein is not intended to take the place of professional medical care; it is not to be used for diagnosing or treating disease; it is not intended to dictate what constitutes reasonable, appropriate or best care for any given health issue; nor is it intended to be used as a substitute for any treatment that may have been prescribed by your doctor. If you have questions regarding a medical condition, always seek the advice of your physician or other qualified health professional.

The reader assumes all responsibility and risk for the use of the information in this book. Under no circumstances shall the author be held liable for any damage resulting directly or indirectly from the information contained herein.

Reference to any products, services, internet links to third parties or other information by trade name, trademark, suppliers, or otherwise does not constitute or imply its endorsement, sponsorship, or recommendation by the author.

Published by Shadow Panther Press
Cover design by www.100covers.com

ISBN: 1093167475
ISBN-13: 978-1093167474

Dedication

This book is dedicated to my Mom, who raised four children and nurtured and supported a family for 60 years. We had a scare back in 2009, when she was diagnosed with breast cancer. We were lucky that her case was not severe or aggressive. Our hope is that she and my Dad will live for many more years. Thanks for everything Mom. I love you.

Table of Contents

About Dr. David Seaman

Dr. Seaman has been studying the relationship between diet and chronic inflammation since 1987. In 2002, he wrote one of the first, if not the absolute first, scientific article that outlined the dietary induction of chronic inflammation:

> Seaman DR. The diet-induced proinflammatory state: a cause of chronic pain and other degenerative diseases? J Manipulative Physiol Ther. 2002;25:168-79.

His scientific papers have been cited by researchers at Harvard Medical School on three occasions, as well as by many researchers at other universities in America, Canada, Brazil, Europe, Russia, Middle East, Africa, India, China, and Australia.

Germane to the subject of this book, the above article about diet-induced inflammation was cited by the following researchers who were investigating diet, inflammation, and breast cancer:

> Ge I, Rudolph A, Shivappa N, et al. Dietary inflammation potential and postmenopausal breast cancer risk in a German case-control study. The Breast. 2015;24:491-96.

> Zahedi H, Djalalinia S, Sadeghi O, et al. Dietary inflammatory potential score and risk of breast cancer: systematic review and meta-analysis. Clin Breast Cancer. 2018;18:e561-e570.

You can follow Dr. Seaman at www.DeFlame.com, as well as at DeFlame Nutrition on YouTube, Facebook, and Instagram, and @DeFlameDoc on Twitter.

Introduction

Approximately 1 out of 8 women will develop breast cancer in their lifetime,[1] making this a highly relevant topic to understand. Almost everyone has been touched by breast cancer, be it a relative or friend. My family is no different. We were fortunate that our mother developed a grade 1 ductal carcinoma that was not invasive, so she is still with us and in her early 80s. Many families have not been so lucky and have lost loved ones much earlier in their lives. My hope is that this book will be widely read so women can prevent the expression of this deadly disease.

The DeFlame Diet for Breast Health and Cancer Prevention is the third in a series of DeFlame books to be published. This is a relatively short book that represents what was going to otherwise be a large chapter in *The DeFlame Diet for Female Health* book, which I plan to publish in 2020.

The first DeFlame book was *The DeFlame Diet* published in 2016, which is the most comprehensive book about diet and inflammation written to date. The second book in the series was *Weight Loss Secrets You Need To Know*. It was published in 2018 and is only $.99 cents for the Kindle book version, so no one with weight management issues should be without it.

The reason why *The DeFlame Diet* approach should be applied to breast health is because all diseases of the breast are pro-inflammatory conditions, the most notable being breast cancer. The relationship between breast cancer and chronic inflammation is mostly unknown by most females in the general population. This book will outline the details for you, which you need to know in order to modify your diet to create a body chemistry environment that is NOT promotional for breast cancer.

References
1. Godet I, Gllkes DM. BRCA1 and BRCA2 mutations and treatment strategies for breast cancer. Integr Cancer Sci Ther. 2017;4: 10.15761/ICST.1000228.

How to read this book

As I mentioned in the introduction, my mother was treated for a grade 1 ductal carcinoma, which is why I asked her to read this book before we went to print. She made two important observations that will likely apply to you. The first observation was that she learned a lot about breast cancer that she did not know and was also never told by her oncologist or primary care physician.

The second observation my mother made was that there were some words and terms that were new to her, which can be frustrating. This is an important issue to address because you will likely encounter some frustration as well…which is totally normal for any of us when we learn something new. It is very important to not let this bother you…you simply need to work through it.

Before I wrote this book, I had collected about 10-15 years worth of information about inflammation and cancer in general, and about inflammation and breast cancer specifically. This means that I worked and struggled through new information for over a decade before writing this book. In other words, you as a reader should expect to encounter new information and new words that you may not understand. If you expect this to be the case, when you encounter some confusion, it will be far less encumbering for your mind, which will allow you to work through it to deepen your understanding about this menacing condition called breast cancer.

Here is an important fact that I have become aware of over the last few decades. People have a misconception about learning. Lots of people think that learning is fun…it is not fun at all; it is frustrating and can even be angering. I remember how I struggled with certain math topics in elementary school, high school, and college – it drove me crazy at times. You probably have a similar memory about the pain of learning, which has continued for me to the present day whenever I begin to learn something new. The actual fun associated with learning happens after you get through the frustration and anger and begin to understand the material. From what I can tell, the frustration and anger associated with learning is the reason why most people tend to avoid learning new material.

My recommendation for you is to work through the material in this book that you find frustrating to learn. Initially, you can skip the information that is new and painful. Go back to it later and spend a little time on the internet acquiring more information to help you learn the new information or language.

By taking this approach, you will gain insight that you did not have previously and also develop a foundation of knowledge to work from. This will help you gain more knowledge and most importantly, help prevent you from being confused by propagandists that benefit from cancer as a business and from others who peddle magical cures.

As you can see on the next page, Chapter 1 outlines the basics of *The DeFlame Diet*. The chapters thereafter outline the inflammatory factors related to breast cancer expression. Armed with the dietary information in Chapter 1, you will be able to visualize and understand how to normalize the various inflammatory factors that promote breast cancer.

Chapter 1
The DeFlame Diet basics

Table 1 below was first published in *The DeFlame Diet* book, which is the most comprehensive book to date that outlines how diet promotes inflammation. The table below outlines pro-inflammatory calories versus *DeFlame Diet* options.

Table 1. Pro-inflammatory vs. DeFlame Diet vs. DeFlame Ketogenic Diet

Pro-inflammatory calories	DeFlame Diet	DeFlame Ketogenic Diet
Refined sugar	Grass-fed meat and wild game	Grass-fed meat and wild game
Refined grains	Meats	Meats
Grain flour products	Wild caught fish	Wild caught fish
Trans fats	Shellfish	Shellfish
Omega-6 seed oils (corn, safflower, sunflower, peanut, etc.)	Chicken	Chicken
	Omega-3 eggs	Omega-3 eggs
	Cheese	Cheese
	Vegetables	Vegetables
	Salads (leafy vegetables)	Salads (leafy vegetables)
	Fruit	* No fruit
	Roots/tubers (potato, yams, sweet potato)	* No roots/tubers
	Nuts (raw or dry roasted)	Nuts (raw or dry roasted)
	Omega-3 seeds: hemp, chia, flax seeds	Omega-3 seeds: hemp, chia, flax seeds
	Dark chocolate	* Sugar free dark chocolate
	Spices of all kinds	Spices of all kinds
	Olive oil, coconut oil, butter, cream, avocado, bacon	Olive oil, coconut oil, butter, cream, avocado, bacon
	Red wine and dark beer	Red wine
	Coffee and tea (green tea is best option)	Coffee and tea (green tea is best option)
		* No legumes and whole grains

Because of the abundance of books, blogs, websites, advertisements, etc., about nutrition, people tend to unnecessarily confuse and complicate how they view a healthy diet. Please notice in Table 1 the list of pro-inflammatory calories, which have no nutritional value; they only serve as a source of calories. Almost 60% of the average American's diet comes from these pro-inflammatory calories, which are implicated in the expression of all chronic diseases, including breast cancer.

The guiding principle behind *The DeFlame Diet* is to normalize all the markers of inflammation, which are outlined in detail in Chapter 9 of *The DeFlame Diet* book. This means that one should not choose their foods based on an ideology, but rather based on your own biochemical needs and food preferences.

The first anti-inflammatory dietary need that applies to EVERYONE is a proper caloric balance. Overeating is the key pro-inflammatory dietary factor to avoid. No matter if one eats a vegan, omnivore, carnivore, Paleo, or ketogenic diet, calories can be over-consumed, which means that all of these diets can be pro-inflammatory. Conversely, if the caloric balance is proper, all of these diets can be anti-inflammatory. This is an especially important concept to understand, as overeating calories leads to obesity, and the pro-inflammatory state of obesity leads to a significant increased risk of expressing breast cancer, which will be discussed in more detail in the obesity chapter of this book.

The challenge people have with giving up pro-inflammatory calories is that they taste really good and we crave them, which is why I use the term "dietary crack" to describe so-called "foods" made from sugar, flour, salt, and omega-6 oils. Breads, cakes, desserts, pretzels, donuts, French fries (and other deep-fried foods), cereals, etc., are the most notable caloric culprits to be avoided. The easiest way to DeFlame your diet is to replace these calories with vegetation, which rapidly leads to a normalization of all inflammatory markers.

The DeFlame Diet book is very inexpensive, at $9.99 for the Kindle book and $24.95 for paperback version.

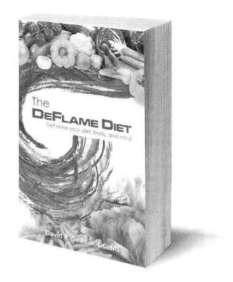

With the above information in mind, it should be understood that it is the cumulative effect of an excess consumption of the pro-inflammatory dietary factors that is the key issue. Eating a cookie every day at 100-200 calories would be irrelevant for the average person if all other pro-inflammatory factors in the diet were eliminated.

There is also a slippery slope to avoid at all costs that needs to be understood. People can maintain proper body weight on a diet of just French fries and donuts. In fact, you can be 100 pounds overweight and go on a 1000 calorie per day diet of just French fries and donuts and achieve a normal body weight. In this extreme case, you would achieve or maintain a normal body weight; however, you would be inflamed by an excess of omega-6 fatty acids from the oils used to make the French fries and donuts, as well as a lack of omega-3 fatty acids, magnesium, polyphenols/carotenoids, and other vitamins and minerals. The goal, as stated above, is to replace pro-inflammatory refined sugar, flour, and oil calories with vegetation.

Chapter 2

How we know breast cancer is an inflammatory disease

We now know that all cancers, not just breast cancer, are inflammatory diseases. Multiple studies have outlined this over the past several years. However, the relationship between inflammation and cancer was first hypothesized over 150 years ago. Consider this introductory statement from an article published in 2002.[1]

"The functional relationship between inflammation and cancer is not new. In 1863, Virchow hypothesized that the origin of cancer was at sites of chronic inflammation, in part based on his hypothesis that some classes of irritants, together with the tissue injury and ensuing inflammation they cause, enhance cell proliferation."

"Recent data have expanded the concept that inflammation is a critical component of tumor progression. Many cancers arise from sites of infection, chronic irritation and inflammation. It is now becoming clear that the tumor microenvironment, which is largely orchestrated by inflammatory cells, is an indispensable participant in the neoplastic [cancerous] process, fostering proliferation, survival and migration [of tumors]."

If you want more evidence that cancer is an inflammatory state or disease, all you need to do is an internet search with the terms, cancer and inflammation, and multiple articles will appear.[2-7] Less articles will appear if you search specifically for breast cancer, or other specific cancers, and inflammation.

With the above in mind, scientists made a definitive statement at the end of 2010 about inflammation and breast cancer that should be understood, which was reported in ScienceDaily on December 15, 2010, in an article entitled, "Breast inflammation is key to cancer growth, researchers say." The scientists identified that the nuclear factor kappa-B (NF-kB) inflammation signaling pathway is a key linchpin in driving breast cancer.[7]

They also found that by blocking NF-kB, they were able to block the onset and progression of breast cancer in living animals. This means that you should know a little about NF-kB, which was outlined in non-complicated language with multiple images in Chapter 9 of *The DeFlame Diet* book. On the next page is a modified image for this book so you can conceptualize how NF-kB works to "flame us up" to promote cancer.

The basic way to view NF-kB is that it functions like a smoke alarm in your house. Indeed, consider the title of this article:

> Ahn KS, Aggarwal BB. Transcription factor NF-kB: a sensor for smoke and stress signals. Ann NY Acad Sci. 2005;1056:218-33.

NF-kB senses alterations in, and challenges to, normal physiology and then mounts an inflammation response to deal with the problem. The modern day issue that we must contend with is the fact that most people adopt a pro-inflammatory lifestyle that chronically activates NF-kB, so that people live in a chronically activated inflammatory state that leads to the develop of cancer and other chronic diseases, including chronic pain and depression.

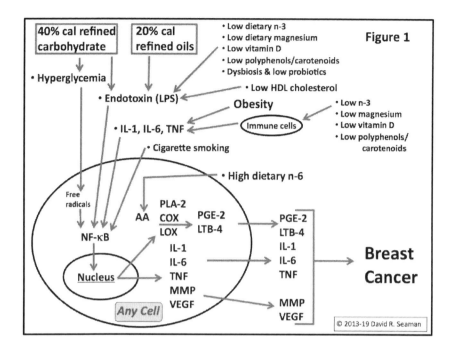

Figure 1

As mentioned above, each of the steps in this image are described in detail in *The DeFlame Diet* book, which includes 9 different pictures that show the progression steps associated with the various pro-inflammatory stimulators of NF-kB.

The primary dietary problem that underpins all chronic diseases is the over consumption of refined carbohydrates (sugar and flour products) and omega-6 (n-6) oils, which make up almost 60% of the average American's calories. These fake "foods" lack key DeFlaming nutrients, the most notable being omega-3 fatty acids, magnesium, and polyphenols/carotenoids (the anti-inflammatory pigments found in vegetation). Sun-avoidance or too much sunscreen leads to vitamin D deficiency.

A lack of omega-3s, magnesium, polyphenols/carotenoids, and vitamin D promotes gut bacteria dysfunction (dysbiosis/low probiotics), which allows for the greater absorption of pro-inflammatory endotoxin/LPS from gut bacteria, which then activates NF-kB. The same deficiencies cause immune cells throughout the body to release their pro-inflammatory cytokines (IL-1, IL-6, TNF), which also stimulate NF-kB.

After several years of overeating refined sugar, flour, and oils, women become obese. There are two primary cell types in fat tissue, those being adipocytes (fat cells) and immune cells. The body of lean people contains "lean" fat cells and anti-inflammatory immune cells that release anti-inflammatory and healing chemicals (adiponectin, IL-10, arginase). In contrast, the body fat of obese people contains "obese" fat cells and pro-inflammatory immune cells, which release pro-inflammatory cytokines (IL-1, IL-6, TNF), which also stimulate NF-kB.

Part of the obesity development process involves a reduction in circulating levels of anti-inflammatory HDL cholesterol. This is highly problematic, as HDL cholesterol functions to normally antagonize and remove the endotoxin/LPS that we are normally exposed to. Without adequate HDL, this will allow endotoxin/LPS levels to rise abnormally, which further stimulates NF-kB. If you happen to also be a smoker, this serves as another stimulator of NF-kB and breast cancer promotion.[8]

After being stimulated, NF-kB moves into the nucleus of the cell, which leads to the production of up to 400 different inflammatory chemicals,[9] of which only seven are listed in Figure 1. It is not important that you recognize or understand the various inflammatory chemicals (PGE-2, LTB-4, IL-1, IL-6, TNF, MMP, and VEGF), some of which will be discussed in future chapters. For now, you just need to know that these are some of the many chemicals that promote and characterize breast cancer and other chronic diseases.

Note also in Figure 1, that NF-kB signaling is occurring in a cell named "any cell." The reason for this is that all cells can produce inflammatory chemicals when exposed to the various pro-inflammatory dietary choices. In the case of breast cancer, the primary cells involved include fibroblasts, immune cells, and the epithelial cells that line the milk-forming lobules and ducts of the mammary gland. It is the epithelial cells that become cancerous. The breast also contains fat cells, which "flame up" during the obesity state and participate in the local inflammation that promotes cancer.[10-12]

The proper concept to understand regarding inflammation and cancer is the cumulative nature of the dietary inflammatory burden to which one is exposed. Notice that all the arrows in Figure 1 lead to the activation of NF-kB. This means that multiple aspects of a pro-inflammatory diet drive NF-kB production, which is a primary driver of chronic inflammation. In the context of this book, we know for sure that NF-kB is an active player in most human cancers, including the breast.[13,14] In one animal model, the scientists discovered that the NF-kB pathway governed the breast cancer process.[7]

Not surprisingly, animal models have demonstrated that caloric restriction can reduce tumor growth by reducing the activity of NF-kB.[15] This is especially beneficial if sugar, flour, and oil calories are replaced with vegetation, which is rich in anti-inflammatory pigments called polyphenols and carotenoids. It is these pigments that exert an NF-kB inhibitory effect, which down-regulates the cancerous process.[16]

References

1. Coussens LM, Werb Z. Inflammation and cancer. Nature. 2002;420:860-67.
2. DeNardo DG, Coussens LM. Inflammation and breast cancer. Balancing immune response: crosstalk between adaptive and innate immune cells during breast cancer progression. Breast Cancer Res. 2007;9(4):212.
3. Cole SW. Chronic inflammation and breast cancer recurrence. J Clin Oncol. 2009;27:3418-19.
4. Korkaya H, Kim G, Davis A, et al. Activation of an IL-6 inflammatory loop mediates trastuzumab resistance in HER2+ breast cancer by expanding the cancer stem cell population. Mol Cell. 2012;47:1-15.
5. Multhoff G, Molls M, Radons J. Chronic inflammation and cancer development. Front Immunol. 2012;2:1-17.
6. Agnoli C, Grioni S, Pala V, et al. Biomarkers of inflammation and breast cancer risk: a case-control study nested in the EPIC-Varese cohort. Sci Reports. 2017;7:12708.

7. Liu M, Sakamaki T, Casimiro MC et al. The canonical NF-kB pathway governs mammary tumorigenesis in transgenic mice and tumor cell expansion. Cancer Res. 2010;70:10464-73.

8. Kispert S, McHowat J. Recent insights into cigarette smoking as a lifestyle risk factor for breast cancer. Breast Cancer – Targets Ther. 2017;9:127-32.

9. Ahn KS, Aggarwal BB. Transcription factor NF-kB: a sensor for smoke and stress signals. Ann NY Acad Sci. 2005;1056:218-33.

10. Vaysse C, Lomo J, Garred O, et al. Inflammation of mammary adipose tissue occurs in overweight and obese patients exhibiting early-stage breast cancer. NPJ Breast Cancer. 2017;3:19.

11. Morris PG, Hudis CA, Giri D, et al. Inflammation and increased aromatase expression occur in the breast tissue of obese women with breast cancer. Cancer Prev Res. 2011;4:1021-29.

12. Jee J, Hong BS, Ryu HS, et al. Transition into inflammatory cancer-associated adipocytes in breast cancer microenvironment requires microRNA regulatory mechanism. PLoS ONE. 2017;12(3): e0174126.

13. Van Waes C. Nuclear factor-kB in development, prevention, and therapy of cancer. Clin Cancer Res. 2007;13:1076-82.

14. Xia Y, Shen S, Verma IM. NF-kB, an active player in human cancers. Cancer Immunol Res. 2014;2:823-30.

15. Mulrooney TJ, Marsh J, Urits I, Seyfried TN, Mukherjee P. Influence of caloric restriction on constitutive expression of NF-kB in an experimental mouse astrocytoma. PLoS ONE. 2011;6(3):e18985.

16. Gupta SC, Kim JH, Kannappan R, et al. Role of nuclear factor-k-B-mediated inflammatory pathways in cancer-related symptoms and their regulation by nutritional agents. Exp Biol Med. 2011;236:658-71.

Chapter 3
Understanding the BRCA (estrogen) gene and breast cancer

The BRCA genes (BRCA 1 and BRCA 2) are the most understood genes that increase one's risk for developing breast cancer. BRCA is the acronym for BReast (BR) and CAncer (CA).

The BRCA gene made headlines when notable actresses (Angelina Joli and Christina Applegate) had elective double mastectomies in order to prevent the emergence of breast cancer. Christina Applegate also had her ovaries and fallopian tubes removed because the BRCA gene mutation is also associated with an increased risk of ovarian cancer.

It turns out that only 5% of all breast cancers occur in women with the BRCA gene mutation,[1,2] which means that 95% of all breast cancers do NOT involve the mutation. However, recent estimates suggest that 55% to 65% of BRCA1 mutation carriers, and approximately 45% of BRCA2 mutation carriers will develop breast cancer by age 70.[2] While this is alarming, we should also appreciate that this means approximately 50% of BRCA mutation carriers will *never* develop breast cancer.

A recent study of 1504 patients with BRCA1 or BRCA2 mutations showed a reduced risk of 50% for developing contralateral breast cancer when taking tamoxifen to suppress secondary tumor formation.[1] What is tamoxifen?

Tamoxifen is an estrogen receptor blocker, which inhibits estrogen from binding to the breast cancer cell and stimulating its growth. Arimidex is a drug that inhibits an enzyme called aromatase, which is involved in the synthesis of estrogen. Any woman with breast cancer will be tested to see if her cancer cells are estrogen positive, which means that cancer cells grow in response to the hormone estrogen. If her cancer is estrogen positive, she will likely be prescribed Arimidex, to inhibit aromatase, or Tamoxifen to inhibit the estrogen receptor.

We can use Arimidex biochemistry to understand how diet can influence the BRCA gene, whether you have the mutation or not. In short, a pro-inflammatory diet can influence the BRCA gene to become inhibited and no longer protective against breast cancer expression. Here is how this works…

One of the ways that BRCA inhibits breast cancer expression is by inhibiting the synthesis of estrogen. In short, a properly acting BRCA gene inhibits the aromatase gene from overproducing estrogen. This mechanism is outlined in Figure 1. Notice that there are two stimulators and the BRCA inhibitor for the aromatase gene, which allows for the proper balance of estrogen production.

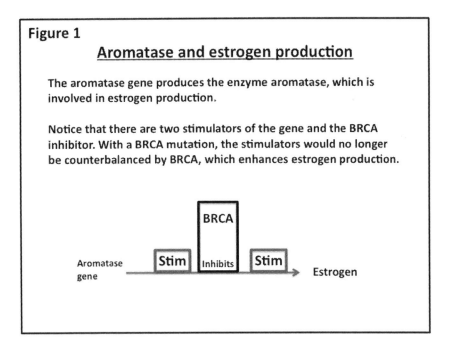

Figure 1
Aromatase and estrogen production

The aromatase gene produces the enzyme aromatase, which is involved in estrogen production.

Notice that there are two stimulators of the gene and the BRCA inhibitor. With a BRCA mutation, the stimulators would no longer be counterbalanced by BRCA, which enhances estrogen production.

BRCA

Aromatase gene   Stim Inhibits Stim   Estrogen

It turns out that a very specific source of dietary inflammation is capable of both inhibiting the BRCA gene and activating the stimulators of the aromatase gene to promote cancer. The dietary issue for this is an excess of omega-6 fatty acids. *The DeFlame Diet* book contains over 60 pages devoted to fats/lipids, so I will refer you to my first book for the details that includes pictures of omega-3, omega-6, omega-9, saturated fats, and trans fatty acids.

In short, the omega-3 and omega-6 fatty acids are the most important regulators of inflammation. The omega-3s are anti-inflammatory and the omega-6s are mostly pro-inflammatory. We need small amounts of each and an equal balance between the two. In fact, for thousands of years, humans consumed a diet that was balanced between omega-6s (n-6) and omega-3s (n-3). The ideal n-6 to n-3 ratio is 1:1. The operational goal should be at least better than 4:1. The problem we have in America is that our n-6 to n-3 ratio is 10:1 to as bad as greater than 25:1.

The source of excess omega-6 fatty acids in the modern diet are specific oils, the most notable and commonly consumed being corn, safflower, sunflower, cottonseed, peanut, and soybean oils. The vast major of fatty acids in these oils are omega-6. These are the oils found in nearly all packaged foods and deep-fried foods. Potato chips, for example, derive most of their calories from the omega-6 oils they are cooked in.

After eating these oiled foods, the human body converts the omega-6 linoleic acid into another omega-6 called arachidonic acid. We also get an abnormal dose of arachidonic acid when we eat meat, fish, and chicken that have been fed a diet of grains, which contain only omega-6 fatty acids and no omega-3 fatty acids at all.

The arachidonic acid that we make from omega-6 oils and get directly from grain-fed animals is then converted into prostaglandin E2, which is highly pro-inflammatory when produced in excess. In Figure 2 below, notice that PGE2 inhibits BRCA and activates the stimulators of the aromatase gene to overproduce estrogen.

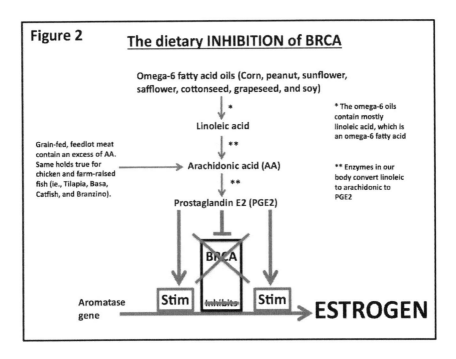

Look again real quick at Figure 1 in Chapter 2. Notice that approximately 20% of the calories consumed by Americans come from refined omega-6 oils. Before the modern era, we ate corn, peanuts, and soybeans, but *never* ever consumed the pure oil from corn, peanuts, soybeans, safflower seeds, and sunflower seeds. By eating these omega-6 oils in substantial quantities, woman dramatically alter their body's fatty acid balance in favor of an overproduction of PGE2, which powerfully stimulates the production of estrogen and mimics a BRCA mutation.

It should not be surprising that 95% of breast cancer sufferers do not have the actual BRCA mutation, but instead they have the "functional mutation" created by overeating omega-6 oils, which leads to the inhibition of BRCA. In fact, it turns out that PGE2 is the most potent stimulator of estrogen production in the human body.[3] Estrogen is mostly produced in the ovaries; however, part of the breast cancer growth process involves the production of estrogen within the breast itself, referred to below as the local production of estrogen.

As stated in the previous chapter, the primary cells involved in breast cancer expression are fibroblasts, immune cells, and the malignant breast epithelial cells. It is the breast tissue fibroblasts that are stimulated by PGE2 to produce aromatase and estrogen locally in the breast, which is a requirement for cancerous breast epithelial cells to grow and become immortalized. In a non-cancerous state, fibroblasts will normally differentiate into mature fat cells that do not produce estrogen. It turns out that pro-inflammatory cytokines, such as TNF and interleukin-11 (IL-11) prevent the maturation of breast estrogen-producing fibroblasts into non-estrogen-producing fat cells.[3]

If you take a quick look at Figure 1 in Chapter 2, you will notice that multiple pro-inflammatory dietary choices lead to an increased production of TNF. The last thing a woman should do is eat in a fashion that increases TNF, which can suppress the maturation of estrogen-producing breast fibroblasts into non-estrogen-producing fat cells. As this unfortunate process develops, the malignant epithelial cells that emerge will locally secrete both TNF and IL-11, which further suppresses nearby fat cell maturation to ensure a constant supply of produced estrogen.[3]

About 80% of all breast cancers are estrogen-receptor positive, which means that estrogen is stimulatory to breast cancer expression, which has been the scenario described thus far, which addresses the vast majority of individuals. In contrast, estrogen-receptor negative breast cancer, which accounts for approximately 20% of cases, does not require an estrogen stimulus for the cancer to proliferate.

Whether breast cancer is estrogen-receptor positive or negative, both are still pro-inflammatory states that desperately need a DeFlaming lifestyle. Basic factors that typically characterize women who develop estrogen-positive breast cancer is low parity (number of times a pregnancy has been carried beyond 20 weeks), late age of first birth, and early age of menarche (the first menstrual period). The predictors for estrogen-negative breast cancer include low socioeconomic status, poor diet (excess sugar, flour, and refined oil intake), and early age of menarche.[4] The average age of menarche is 12-13 years.

As early menarche is common to both estrogen+ and estrogen- breast cancers, we should understand what leads to an earlier than expected first menstrual period. Not surprisingly, one of the most robust predictors is abdominal body fat accumulation,[5] which is an easily modifiable risk factor. Exposure to certain environmental chemicals, such as pthalates (plasticizers) and polychlorinated biphenyls, have been associated with earlier breast development and menarche.[5] Both obesity and environment chemicals will be discussed in more detail in their respective chapters in this book.

The obvious choice to make, no matter if your decision is to prevent breast cancer or deal with estrogen-positive or estrogen-negative cancer, is to absolutely eliminate all refined sugar, flour, and omega-6 oils from the diet. This DeFlaming approach should be done as a family-plan for overall health promotion; not just because of breast cancer risk or diagnosis. This is an entire family issue. Heart disease, Alzheimer's disease, osteoarthritis, depression, all cancers, menstrual pain, acne, and most other chronic diseases are pushed into expression by the overconsumption of refined sugar, flour, and omega-6 oils. So, the entire family should be committed to avoiding these highly inflammatory calories, which will likely cause problems for other family members over time.

References

1. Godet I, Gllkes DM. BRCA1 and BRCA2 mutations and treatment strategies for breast cancer. Integr Cancer Sci Ther. 2017;4: 10.15761/ICST.1000228.
2. van der Groep P, van der Wall E, van Diest PJ. Pathology of hereditary breast cancer. Cell Oncol. 2011;34:71-88.
3. Bulun SE, Lin Z, Zhao H, et al. Regulation of aromatase expression in breast cancer tissue. Ann NY Acad Sci. 2009;1155:121-31.
4. Hidaka BH, Boddy AM. Estrogen receptor negative breast cancer risk is associated with a fast life history strategy. Evol Med Pub Health. 2016(1):17-20.

5. Karapanou O, Papdimitriou A. Determinants of menarche. Reprod Biol Endocrinol. 2010;8:115.

Chapter 4
Gingival and periodontal disease and breast cancer risk

I have spoken at several dental conventions in the last few years. There are groups of dentists that are deeply concerned about the relationship between oral and systemic (full body) health. The most notable dental group I am aware of that is devoted to this topic is the American Academy of Oral and Systemic Health (AAOSH). Many members of the American Academy of Craniofacial Pain are also very active in promoting anti-inflammatory nutrition to their patients.

I included this short chapter because more and more is being discovered about how poor dental health is not just a local problem; it leads to chronic systemic inflammation. Multiple diseases have been linked to gingival and periodontal disease,[1] such as heart disease,[2] depression,[3] diabetes,[4] Alzheimer's disease,[5] and various cancers including the breast.[6]

It is not uncommon to read and hear that eating fat, especially animal fat, is the cause of chronic disease. This is a grossly oversimplified statement, especially in light of what we know about the traditional arctic circle (Eskimo) diet, which was mostly fatty meats during the winter months. These people did not suffer from an increased risk of any chronic disease due to their fatty meat diets. In fact, traditional Eskimos were a robustly healthy population of people. This fact has been muffled by the misinformation spread by radical vegans who believe that meat eating causes disease.

The first dentist I am aware of that travelled the earth and examined the dental health of various populations was Dr. Weston Price. He wrote a book about his travels during the 1930s entitled, *Nutrition and Physical Degeneration*, which was first published in 1945, and is still available today if you have an interest in reading it. He described the dentition of traditional Eskimos to be almost completely free of cavities. Dr. Price made the following conclusion in his chapter on the Eskimos:

> "Notwithstanding the very inhospitable part of the world in which they reside, with nine or ten months of winter and only two or three months of summer, and in spite of the absence for long periods of plant foods and dairy products and eggs, the Eskimos were able to provide their bodies with all the mineral and vitamin requirements from sea foods, stored greens and berries and plants from the sea."

All of this changed as the traditional Eskimo diet became "westernized" which means they became "refined sugared, floured, and oiled" over time. Dr. Price noticed this in the 1930s, as did other scientists. For example, Dr. Rabinowitch, a Canadian researcher, studied the Canadian Eskimos in the Eastern Arctic.[7] Part of his assessment of "westernization" of the Eskimo diet involved the use of flour in their diets. Those Eskimos who ate a lot of flour, and still had their teeth cleaned by dentists, were far more likely to have cavities and other health issues compared to the Eskimos eating the traditional diet. As Rabinowitch travelled further north, wherein flour was rare, and Eskimos ate their traditional diets, they were found to be much more physically healthy in general and had substantially less cavities. I want to emphasize that Eskimos eating the traditional diet that is rich in fatty sea and land animals, and free of refined sugar, flour, and oils, is NOT associated with breast cancer or any other cancer.[8] However, today cancer is on the rise in the Eskimo population and this appears to be due to a drastic change in dietary pattern and exposure to xenobiotic agents (environmental pollutants).[9] Xenoestrogens will be discussed in Chapter 6.

It should be obvious from this Eskimo example that refined sugar, flour, and oils are the problematic pro-inflammatory calories that need to be drastically limited in the diet. When we eat sugar and flour, they are metabolized by bacteria involved in dental biofilm formation, which generates acidic byproducts that can lead to demineralization of the tooth structure.[10] Natural foods like raisins, apples, bananas, and chocolate are rapidly cleared from tooth surfaces; however, adding sugar to these foods leads to increased dental plaque formation. This was demonstrated in a study in children wherein they compared sugared raisin bran cereal to a mix of bran flakes and raisins without sugar.[11]

It is important to understand that dental plaque is actually a bacterial plaque, to which the immune system reacts with an inflammatory reaction. This develops slowly over time, progressing to gingivitis, and eventually periodontitis. This progressive developmental process is associated with increased levels of circulating endotoxin/LPS derived from the dental plaque.[12] Recall that in Chapter 2 of this book, endotoxin/LPS was described as an activator of NF-kB and the subsequent inflammatory process.

People with dental-related endotoxemia, have a commensurate increase in circulating levels of C-reactive protein (CRP),[13] which is the easiest to measure, and most well-known, marker of chronic systemic inflammation. The last thing anyone needs is an elevated CRP level, which is associated with the expression of most chronic diseases, including breast cancer. In fact, elevated levels of CRP are associated with a greater risk of developing breast cancer,[14] and higher and higher levels of CRP at the time of breast cancer diagnosis is associated with a poorer prognosis.[15] CRP is typically viewed as a marker of inflammation; however, we also know that CRP can perpetuate inflammation by stimulating cells to release pro-inflammatory cytokines.[16] CRP and all the other relevant inflammatory markers you should track can be found in Chapter 9 of *The DeFlame Diet* book.

Based on the information in this chapter, we can see that avoidance of refined sugar and flour calories is of paramount concern for the combination of dental and systemic health. We should all have our teeth cleaned regularly by dental professionals and be diligent with our home care, especially flossing, to avoid the progression from plaque formation, to gingivitis, to periodontitis.

Xylitol gum and toothpaste (and other products) are probably the best option for dental care. Xylitol is a polyol, which is a family of sweeteners that actually prevent dental plaque and related decay and inflammation, and have beneficial effects on our gut bacteria.

References

1. Cardoso EM, Reis C, Manzanares-Cespedes MC. Chronic periodontitis, inflammatory cytokines, and interrelationship with other chronic diseases. Postgrad Med. 2018;130:98-104.
2. Dhadse P, Gattani D, Mishra R. The link between periodontal disease and cardiovascular disease: how far have we come in the last two decades? J Indian Soc Periodontol. 2010;14:148-54.
3. Sundararajan S, Muthukumar S, Rao SR. Relationship between depression and chronic periodontitis. J Indian Soc Periodontol. 2015;19:294-96.
4. Mealey BL. Periodontal disease and diabetes. 2006;137(Suppl 2):S26-S31.
5. Abbayya K, Puthanakar NY, Naduwinmani S, Chidambar YS. Association between periodontitis and Alzheimer's disease. N Am J Med Sci. 2015;7:241-46.
6. Sfreddo CS, Maier J, De David SC, Susin C, Moreira CH. Periodontitis and breast cancer: a case-controlled study. Community Dent Oral Epidemiol. 2017;00:1-7.
7. Rabinowitch IM. Clinical and other observations on Canadian Eskimos in the Eastern Arctic. J Canadian Med Assoc. 1936;34:487-501.
8. Friborg JT, Melbye M. Cancer patterns in Inuit populations. Lancet Oncol. 2008;9:892-90.
9. Donaldson SG, Van Oostdam J, Tikhonov C, et al. Environmental contaminants and human health in the Canadian Arctic. Sci Total Environ. 2010;408;5165-234.
10. Gupta P, Gupta N, Pawar AP, et al. Role of sugar and sugar substitutes in dental caries: a review. ISRN Dent. 2013;519421.
11. Utreja A, Lingstrom P, Evans CA, Salzmann LB, Wu CD. The effect of raisin-containing cereals on the pH of dental plaque in young children. Pediatr Dent. 2009;31:498-503.
12. Shaddox LM, Wiedy J, Calderon NL, et al. Local inflammatory markers and system endotoxin in aggressive periodontitis. J Dent Res. 2011;90:1140-44.
13. Podzimek S, Mysak J, Janatova T, Duskova J. C-reactive protein in peripheral blood of patients with chronic and aggressive periodontitis, gingivitis, and gingival recessions. Med Inflamm. 2015: Article ID 564858, pages 1-7.
14. Guo L, Liu S, Zhang S et al. C-reactive protein and risk of breast cancer: a systematic review and meta-analysis. Sci Rep. 2015;5:10508.
15. Allin KH, Nordestgaard BG, Flyger H, Bojesen SE. Elevated pre-treatment levels of plasma C-reactive protein are associated with poor prognosis after breast cancer: a cohort study. Breast Cancer Res. 2011;13R55.
16. Ouchi N, Walsh K. A novel role for adiponectin in the regulation of inflammation. Arterioscler Thromb Vasc Biol. 2008;28:1219-21.

Chapter 5
How sugar consumption compromises mitochondria to promote cancer

If you search the internet, you will see blogs, articles, and videos that talk about how eating sugar causes cancer, or that sugar feeds cancer. This statement needs to be put into perspective, so that the proper amount of concern can be applied to this issue.

The average American consumes 40% of their calories from refined sugar and flour. This amounts to over 100 pounds of consumed refined sugar per year, and probably a similar amount of flour. There is no place for this amount of sugar and flour in the human diet.

When excess sugar and flour products are consumed, they are digested and absorbed, and this leads to substantially elevated levels of circulating blood glucose. When we are young, this initially occurs only after eating. However, as this becomes a habitual eating pattern over time, people develop elevated levels of fasting and postprandial glucose, such that they perpetually live in a hyperglycemic (high glucose) state.

One of the many metabolic changes that occur in cancer cells is a shift towards a reliance on sugar as the fuel for cell energy production and an inability of a cancer cell to make energy from fat and ketones (a fat-like substance). This shift is so profound that cancer cells are said to have a "glucose addiction."[1] The term "Warburg effect" is used to describe the altered energy utilization pattern of cancer cells. It was discovered in the 1920s by Otto Warburg, for which he was awarded the Noble Prize in 1931. The biochemical pathway that is utilized to create energy from this glucose addiction leads to an excessive production of lactic acid, which is why the local tumor environment is acidic.

Figure 1 below illustrates how a normal cell obtains energy from the calories we eat. Normal cells can make energy called adenosine triphosphate (ATP) from glucose, fatty acids (from fat), and ketones, each of which must first be transported from the blood supply into an individual cell. Once inside a cell, via a process called glycolysis, glucose is converted to pyruvate, which is then shuttled into mitochondria, and then converted into acetyl-CoA. Fatty acids and ketones are also transported into mitochondria to be converted into acetyl-CoA. As the arrow indicates, acetyl-CoA is transported into the inner membrane area of the mitochondria where ATP (cell energy is produced). ATP functions in the body in a fashion that is similar to putting gas in the car. For us humans, we make our own gas (ATP) from glucose, fatty acids, and ketones.

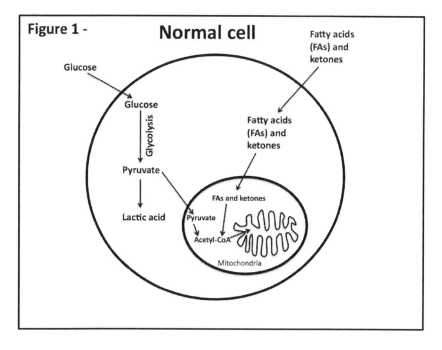

When glucose, fatty acids, and ketones are used for energy in mitochondria, the term oxidation is used. It turns out that oxygen is required by mitochondria to generate ATP from these three substances – which is why this process is called aerobic cellular respiration (or metabolism). When oxygen is not available, we shift to anaerobic metabolism, wherein mitochondria are not actively producing energy. In this situation we can only generate energy (ATP) from glucose via glycolysis, which occurs outside the mitochondria. This glycolytic process also leads to the production of lactic acid, as illustrated in Figure 1.

Notice also in Figure 1 the shape of the inner membrane of the mitochondria into which the acetyl-CoA is transported. It is extremely convoluted, which allows for a large surface in which energy (ATP) can be produced.

One of the most striking differences between normal and cancer cells is the shape of the mitochondria. Figure 2 illustrates a normal cell versus a cancer cell.

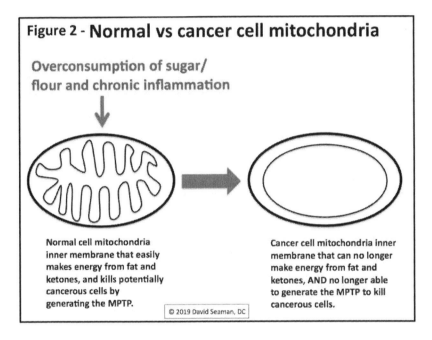

Figure 2 - **Normal vs cancer cell mitochondria**

Overconsumption of sugar/ flour and chronic inflammation

Normal cell mitochondria inner membrane that easily makes energy from fat and ketones, and kills potentially cancerous cells by generating the MPTP.

Cancer cell mitochondria inner membrane that can no longer make energy from fat and ketones, AND no longer able to generate the MPTP to kill cancerous cells.

© 2019 David Seaman, DC

Notice in the normal cell that the inner membrane of the mitochondria is highly convoluted compared to that in a cancer cell that appears oval. The inner membrane of the mitochondria in cancer cells has been mutated and is no longer able to create energy (ATP) from glucose, but more importantly, cancer cells are unable to create energy (ATP) from fat and ketones,[2,3] which is why they are described as being "glucose addicted." This means that cancer cells have to rely on energy production via glycolysis, which involves the conversion of glucose to lactic acid, as illustrated previously in Figure 1. This is why the local cancer tissue environment is so acidic; large amounts of lactic acid are being continuously produced.

On the surface, it may not readily make sense why cancer cells would metabolically "silence" their mitochondria so they become reliant on energy production from glycolysis. The reason has to do with a mostly unknown or forgotten function of mitochondria. Cancer cells must mutate their mitochondria because it is the mitochondria that play a key role in the normal turnover of our body cells. Old cells are replaced with new cells, and this is an ongoing process throughout our lifespan.

This process is called apoptosis, which means "programmed cell death." Mitochondria are able to sense when it is time for the cell to die and they produce what is called the mitochondrial permeability transition pore (MPTP), which leads to cell death.[2-4] Only a normal inner membrane has the capacity to generate the MPTP to kill the cell. Cancer cells lack a normal inner membrane, which prevents MPTP formation, and this allows cancer cells to become "immortalized" and no longer susceptible to apoptosis. Figure 2 illustrates how normal mitochondria are transformed into a cancer cell mitochondria that now evades cell death signaling and becomes an immortalized cancer cell.

Not surprisingly, it is an overconsumption of sugar and flour, coupled with chronic inflammation, that mutates the inner membrane of the mitochondria to one that is no longer able to generate the mitochondrial permeability transition pore, which is needed so that that aging or unhealthy cells can die and be replaced with healthy cells.[2,3]

An additional modification occurs in breast cancer cells, as with other cancer cells, which is also illustrated in Figure 3. Notice the abundance of insulin receptors on the cell membrane of the breast cancer cell compared to the normal cell, a fact that has been known for decades.[5-7] Cancer cells create this mutation in order to allow a much greater absorption of glucose into the cancer cell to fuel its extreme energy and growth demands.

It turns out that estrogen is one of the drivers of this excess incorporation of insulin receptors into the breast cancer cell membrane.[8] Recall from Chapter 3 of this book that refined omega-6 oil consumption leads to an excess of PGE2 synthesis, which promotes estrogen production. You can now appreciate how refined sugar, flour, and oils work together to create breast cancer.

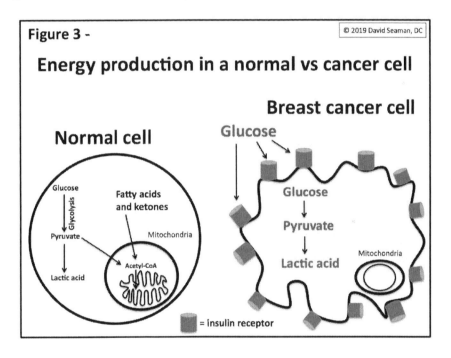

Figure 3 - © 2019 David Seaman, DC

Energy production in a normal vs cancer cell

The problem with overeating sugar is that normal cells take on a metabolic phenotype, or functional state, that resembles the biochemistry of cancer cells.[9,10] This does not mean that normal cells will become cancer cells if you have a couple of donuts and heavily sweetened coffee; but it does suggest that chronically overeating sugar nudges cells in that direction over time and facilitates the transformation of a normal cell into one that is cancerous. In one study that looked at skeletal muscle metabolism in relation to diabetes, subjects were given approximately 140 grams of glucose solution per day for 4 weeks,[10] which amounts to about 40 ounces of cola soda per day. Because an obvious shift in glucose handling by muscles took place so quickly, the authors tell us that the study was limited to 4 weeks due to ethical reasons.

Another pro-cancerous issue needs to be discussed regarding excess sugar and flour consumption. Not only do blood glucose and insulin levels increase after eating sugar, a glucose-related growth factor also becomes elevated, which is called insulin-like growth factor-1 (IGF-1). There are many growth factors involved in cancer expression, and this should not be surprising, as tumors cannot grow in size without being stimulated to do so. Growth factors, like IGF-1 and VEGF, stimulate the growth of tumors. VEGF stands for vascular endothelial growth factor, which is involved in the growth of new blood vessels that are required for tumors to continue growing in size. VEGF is one of the seven inflammatory chemicals in Figure 1 in Chapter 2 that are elevated in people who chronically overeat pro-inflammatory foods.

The combination of excess pro-inflammatory glucose, insulin, IGF-1, cytokines (IL-1, IL-6, TNF), and VEGF, hyper-activate a signaling molecule called mTOR.[11] For our purposes here, it is accurate to describe mTOR as a "proliferaTOR" substance, which means it is a cancer cell growth proliferator.[11-13] Scientists explain that mTOR is almost obligatorily activated in cancer cells,[11] which means we need to do all we can to DeFlame the body so that mTOR activity is properly regulated. In the next chapter, mTOR signaling will be illustrated, but for now, consider the following information.

How milk augments mTOR signaling to promote the cancerous state

Milk is considered to be a low glycemic food, meaning that it does not lead to elevated levels of circulating glucose. However, milk is a potent stimulator of insulin and IFG-1 production, both of which activate mTOR, which suggests that people with cancer or at risk for developing cancer, should be avoiding milk consumption.

A scientist named Dr. Bodo Melnik from the University of Osnabruck in Germany has spent much of his recent research career focusing on the pro-inflammatory issues related to milk consumption – he has published at least 30 scientific papers on this topic. This quote below is from Dr. Melnik [and co-authors] about prostate cancer; however, it can be applied to breast cancer as well, since both cancers are caused, in part, by an induction of mTOR signaling:[14]

> "Paleolithic (anti-inflammatory) diets and restriction of dairy protein intake, especially during mTOR-dependent phases of prostate development and differentiation, may offer protection from the most common dairy-promoted cancer in men of Western societies."

Prostate cancer is the most common dairy-promoted cancer in men, while breast cancer is the most common dairy-promoted cancer in women. Milk consumption leads to exaggerated mTOR signaling in women, men, and children. We incorrectly think of milk as a food, however, it should be properly viewed as a "growth" promoter.

Consider that new-born calves grow massively during the first year of life, not because of eating grass, hay, or grains; it is because of the growth factors in cow's milk for the purpose of helping to rapidly increase the size of a newborn calf. Thereafter, cows and steers naturally eat grass all day. This is why Melnik refers to milk not just as a food but as "a genetic transfection system activating mTORC1 signaling for postnatal growth."[20] In other words, we humans should *not* be consuming a growth factor for baby calves as a staple food in our diets.

Casein is a protein in milk and it increases liver production of IGF-1. In fact, milk consumption elevates blood levels of IGF-1 by 20-30% compared to non-dairy consumers.[15] The whey protein component of milk induces the secretion of a substance called glucose-dependent insulinotropic polypeptide, which stimulates the pancreas to release insulin.[15]

The problem in a nutshell is this. The combination of sugar, flour, and milk represent potent stimulators of insulin and IGF-1, which should absolutely be avoided by those wishing to prevent or manage cancer. This means we should absolutely eliminate the habitual consumption of cookies and milk, cake and milk, bread and milk, cereal and milk, and ice cream from our diets to reduce the inappropriate activation of mTOR.

Starving cancer cells with a ketogenic diet
In April of 2012, Dr. Sanjay Gupta did a piece on this topic for *60 Minutes*, wherein a cancer researcher at Harvard University stated that because of the relationship between sugar and cancer, he simply will not eat sugar.[16] Based on what you just read in this chapter, I am sure that you will agree with this position.

A key dietary goal should be to starve cancer cells of glucose, which means completely avoiding sugar and flour calories. Cancer cells struggle to grow when most of the calories we eat come from fat.

The question is, how far do you wish to take carbohydrate restriction? I think we should all eliminate refined sugar and flour. This can be taken further to move into a state of ketosis. As outlined in Table 1, this requires that the following foods be eliminated from the diet: whole grains, legumes, roots/tubers (i.e., potatoes, sweet potatoes, yams, etc.), and fruit. When we reduce our carbohydrate intake, it forces our liver to make ketones from the fat calories that replaced the carbohydrate calories. This leads to a measurable increase in blood levels of ketones, which is called nutritional ketosis. Below is Table 1 from Chapter 1 that contrasts *The DeFlame Diet* with The DeFlame Ketogenic Diet, so you can see the food options.

Table 1. Pro-inflammatory vs. DeFlame Diet vs. DeFlame Ketogenic Diet

Pro-inflammatory calories	DeFlame Diet	DeFlame Ketogenic Diet
Refined sugar	Grass-fed meat and wild game	Grass-fed meat and wild game
Refined grains	Meats	Meats
Grain flour products	Wild caught fish	Wild caught fish

Trans fats	Shellfish	Shellfish
Omega-6 seed oils (corn, safflower, sunflower, peanut, etc.)	Chicken	Chicken
	Omega-3 eggs	Omega-3 eggs
	Cheese	Cheese
	Vegetables	Vegetables
	Salads (leafy vegetables)	Salads (leafy vegetables)
	Fruit	* No fruit
	Roots/tubers (potato, yams, sweet potato)	* No roots/tubers
	Nuts (raw or dry roasted)	Nuts (raw or dry roasted)
	Omega-3 seeds: hemp, chia, flax seeds	Omega-3 seeds: hemp, chia, flax seeds
	Dark chocolate	* Sugar free dark chocolate
	Spices of all kinds	Spices of all kinds
	Olive oil, coconut oil, butter, cream, avocado, bacon	Olive oil, coconut oil, butter, cream, avocado, bacon
	Red wine and dark beer	Red wine
	Coffee and tea (green tea is best option)	Coffee and tea (green tea is best option)
		* No legumes and whole grains

I think that no more than 100 grams (400 calories) of carbohydrate per day is reasonable for all; however, to get into ketosis, one needs to eat less than 50 grams (200 calories) of carbohydrate per day. If you wish to pursue the ketogenic diet, my recommendation is to get two books written by the leading experts, Drs. Stephen Phinney and Jeff Volek. One is called *The Art and Science of Low Carbohydrate Living* and the other is *The Art and Science of Low Carbohydrate Performance*.

Exogenous ketones (ketone supplements) can be taken as well, which are now readily available to support and maintain the ketosis state. Studies are emerging which demonstrate the utility of ketone supplements in the management of cancer.[17-19] Experimental studies have also demonstrated that ketones help to inhibit inflammation,[20] which is highly desirable, as cancer *is* chronic inflammation.

A final consideration about sugar and breast cancer

"A breast positron emission tomography (PET) scan is an imaging test that uses a radioactive substance (called a tracer) to look for breast cancer. This tracer can help identify areas of cancer that an MRI or CT scan may miss." This is what we are told at Medlineplus, a US government website.[21] We are also told that the tracer is delivered intravenously at the elbow. What we are not told is that the tracer is called fluorodeoxyglucose (FDG)…notice that glucose is part of the tracer. This is because the tracer molecule called ^{18}F is attached to a glucose molecule.

Because FDG is similar to glucose, it is metabolized by the glycolysis pathway, which was discussed earlier in this chapter. This means that the glycolysis-dependent breast cancer cells will suck up FDG, just like glucose from eating sugar and flour, and this will appear as a hotspot on the PET scan due to the accumulation of ^{18}F in the tumor.

Of all the women I have spoken with who have had PET scans performed, none of them were told that it would be a good idea to eliminate refined sugar and flour intake to avoid the calories that breast cancer cells need to grow. These women were angered to find this out from me, rather than from their oncologists or personal physicians.

References

1. Klement RJ, Fink MK. Dietary and pharmacological modification of the insulin/IGF-1 system: exploiting the full repertoire against cancer. Oncogenesis. 2016 Feb 15;5:e193.
2. Seyfried TN, Flores RE, Poff AM, D'Agostino DP. Cancer as a metabolic disease: implications for novel therapeutics. Carcinogenesis. 2014;35:515-27.
3. Seyfried TN. Cancer as a mitochondrial metabolic disease. Front Cell Developmental Biol. 2015;3:43/
4. Regula KM, Ens K, Kirshenbaum LA. Mitochondria-assisted cell suicide: a license to kill. J Mol Cell Cardiol. 2003;35:559-67.
5. Papa V, Pezzino V, Costantino A, et al. Elevated insulin receptor content in human breast cancer. J Clin Invest. 1990;86:1503-10.
6. Milazzo G, Giorgino F, Damante G, et al. Insulin receptor expression and function in human breast cancer. Cancer Res. 1992;52:3924-30.

7. Chan JY, Hackel BJ, Yee D. Targeting insulin receptor in breast cancer using small engineered protein scaffolds. Mol Cancer Therapeutics. 2017;16:1324-341

8. Molloy CA, May FE, Westley BR. Insulin receptor substrate-1 expression is upregulated by estrogen in the MCF-7 human breast cancer cell line. J Biol Chem. 2000;275:12565-71.

9. Onodera Y, Nam JM, Bissell MJ. Increased sugar uptake promotes oncogenesis via EPAC/RAP1 and O-GlcNAc pathways. J Clin Invest. 2014;124(1):367-84.

10. Sartor F, Jackson MJ, Squillace C, et al. Adaptive metabolic response to 4 weeks of sugar-sweetened beverage consumption in healthy, lightly active individuals and chronic high glucose availability in primary human myotubes. Eur J Nutr. 2013;52(3):937-48.

11. Blagosklonny MV. TOR-centric view on insulin resistance and diabetic complications: perspective for endocrinologists and gerontologists. Cell Death Disease. 2013;4:e964.

12. Cargnello M, Tcherkezian J, Roux PP. The expanding role of mTOR in cancer cell growth and proliferation. Mutagenesis. 2015;30:169-76.

13. Laplante M, Sabatini DM. mTOR signaling and growth control and disease. Cell. 2012;149:274-93.

14. Melnick BC, John SM, Carrero-Bastos P, Cordain L. The impact of cow's milk-mediated mTORC1-signalling in the initiation and progression of prostate cancer. Nutr Metab. 2012;9(10:74.

15. Melnick BC. Milk is not just a food but most likely a genetic transfection system activating mTORC1 signalling for postnatal growth. Nutr J. 2013;12:103.

16. 60 Minutes. Dr. Sanjay Gupta reporting the on the disease-driving nature of refined sugar. http://www.cbsnews.com/video/watch/?id=7403942n; https://www.youtube.com/watch?v=aIc6iF5k9v4

17. Poff A, Ari C, Arnold P, Seyfried TN, D'Agostino D. Ketone supplementation decreases tumor cell viability and prolongs survival of mice with metastatic cancer. Int J Cancer. 2014;135:1711-20.

18. Poff AM, Ward N, Seyfried TN, Arnold P, D'Agostino DP. Non-toxic metabolic management of metastatic cancer in VM mice: novel combination of ketogenic diet, ketone suppelmentation, and hyperbaric oxygen therapy. PLoS One. 2015;10(6):e0127407.

19. Poff A, Kesl S, Ward N, D'Agostino D. Metabolic effects of exogenous ketone supplementation – an alternative or adjuvant to the ketogenic diet as a cancer therapy. FASEB J. 2016;30(Suppl 1):Abstract.

20. Youm YH, Nguyen KY, Grant RW, et al. Ketone body B-hydroxybutyrate blocks the NLRP3 inflammasome-mediated inflammatory disease. Nat Med. 2015;21:263-69.

21. https://medlineplus.gov/ency/article/007469.htm

Chapter 6
Xenoestrogens and breast cancer

The term xenobiotic refers to a man-made chemical that is foreign to the human body and to our ecological system; in common language, they are environment pollutants. Xenoestrogens are those foreign chemicals that have an estrogenic effect, which means they elevate estrogen production within the human body, which is clearly promotional of breast cancer and other estrogen-mediated diseases, the most notable being ovarian cancer and endometriosis.

Some people have become exceptionally over-concerned about xenobiotic agents, believing that if it were not for the presence of these substances, conditions like cancer would be unlikely. This view is incorrect. People developed cancer before the days when xenobiotics were more plentiful, so we need a more balanced view. The fact of the matter is that xenobiotics can absolutely promote cancer to some degree and we cannot completely avoid xenobiotic agents.

CDC (Centers for Disease Control) researchers found measurable levels of many phthalate (plasticizers) metabolites in the general population. This finding indicates that phthalate exposure is widespread in the U.S. population. Research has found that adult women have higher levels of urinary metabolites than men for those phthalates that are used in soaps, body washes, shampoos, cosmetics, and similar personal care products.[1]

The issue is that everyone is exposed to xenobiotic agents, but only 1 out of 8 women in their lifetime will develop breast cancer.[2] For men, the number is 1 out of 1000. Obviously, it would be much better if that was also the risk for women. My point is that despite an essentially universally equal exposure to environmental pollutants that we have no control over, there is only 1 in 8 women who will develop breast cancer. So, we cannot look at xenobiotics as the primary problem. I think it is better to understand what it is about the 7 out of 8 women who do NOT get breast cancer, despite a generally similar exposure pattern to xenobiotics in air, water, and food. The two primary risk modifiers are most likely genetics and lifestyle choices. We can obviously not change our genes, but we can certainly change our lifestyle.

Multiple studies have been done that have described the estrogenic and related cancerous effects of personal care products.[3-7] As stated above, xenoestrogens are found in skin moisturizers, sunscreens, deodorants, antiperspirants, makeup, and shampoos. They are also found in plastic, which is why they are commonly called plasticizers, which means if you want to be completely sure you are getting no xenoestrogens in your water, you need to use a glass drinking bottle or a xenoestrogen-free plastic bottle.

I have chosen to not compile a thorough list of potential personal care products containing xenoestrogens. The main reason is that the list is long and I could easily miss many products, which could give a woman the false sense of security that her products are xenoestrogen-free. This means that you need to identify for yourself that the products you use are absolutely free of xenoestrogens. The easiest way to do this is to do an internet search for hormone/xenoestrogen-free products. Here are examples of search terms you can use: hormone-free makeup, hormone-free shampoo, hormone-free moisturizers, hormone-free sunscreen, estrogen-free makeup, estrogen-free shampoo, estrogen-free moisturizers, and estrogen-free sunscreen. You could also use the term xenoestrogen-free and then include the various products. By doing this, you can clear your personal environment of estrogenic products.

Figure 1 on the next page was designed to help orient our thinking in relation to xenoestrogens and lifestyle choices that can support or prevent inappropriate estrogenic activity. The key players in Figure 1 are mTOR and p53. Notice below mTOR it says "The ProliferaTOR." This is because mTOR is described as "master regulator of cell growth and metabolism."[8] The term mTOR translates into mammalian target of rapamycin, which means that the drug rapamycin was identified first and its experimental use was related to a reduction of growth and metabolism.

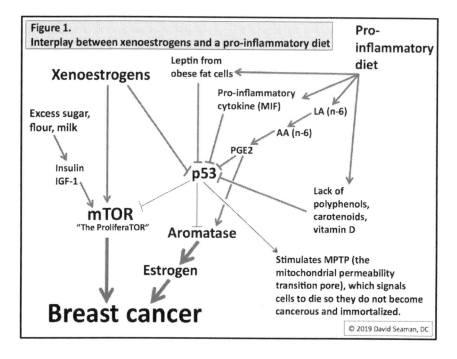

First, it should be understood that mTOR signaling is needed when cell growth is desired; however, mTOR should then be turned off. Consider, for example, that mTOR is involved in the process of muscle mass accumulation with resistance exercise. In fact, mTOR is described as a key regulator in maintaining skeletal muscle mass.[9] This means that we do not want to completely block mTOR; we need to create a biochemical environment in our bodies, wherein mTOR turns on and off properly. In the case of chronic inflammation and worse, as in cancer, mTOR is inappropriately and chronically overactive.

Notice in Figure 1 that xenoestrogens stimulate mTOR.[6] The same holds true for an excess production of estrogen in the body, a process that was outlined in Chapter 3 about the BRCA gene. In Figure 1 above, notice that a pro-inflammatory diet stimulates mTOR, and this is because a pro-inflammatory diet can increase the production of estrogen (see Chapter 3). In Chapter 5, I explained how a pro-inflammatory diet stimulates the production of insulin and IGF-1, both of which also activate mTOR. Between xenoestrogen exposure and a pro-inflammatory diet, mTOR receives an excess of stimulation. The problem is, as Figure 1 illustrates, these same two stimulators also INHIBIT a very important inhibitor of mTOR activity, called p53.[7]

Notice above in Figure 1 that p53 has three very important functions; to inhibit aromatase and estrogen, to inhibit mTOR, and to promote the activation of the mitochondrial permeability transition pore (MPTP),[10-12] which is needed to kill old senescent cells before they become cancerous. Recall that MPTP was described in Chapter 5 in some detail.

Notice also in Figure 1 that the inhibitory arrows going from p53 to mTOR, MPTP and aromatase are small and faintly colored, compared to the bold arrows that simultaneously stimulate mTOR and inhibit p53. This is to reflect how xenoestrogens and a pro-inflammatory diet work together to create a robust pro-inflammatory state that stimulates mTOR and inhibits p53. By inhibiting p53, "the brakes are removed" from mTOR and aromatase, allowing for inappropriate excess of proliferative activity. We need proper p53 activity and poor dietary choices lead to a loss of proper p53 regulation of cancer expression.

Figure 1 highlights three ways in which a pro-inflammatory diet can inhibit p53 and thereby stimulate cancer. Leptin (to be discussed in Chapter 8) and MIF are overproduced in obesity. A lack of polyphenols, carotenoids and vitamin D are related to specific lifestyle choices that typically correlate to the overconsumption of refined sugar, flour, and oils.

Macrophage MIF (migration inhibitory factor) is an inflammatory regulator (cytokine), which is overproduced during obesity and is directly associated with the degree of peripheral insulin resistance and related elevations in blood glucose levels,[13] which means the excess production of MIF is directly related to a pro-inflammatory diet and sedentary living. Increasing evidence suggests that MIF is released by adipose tissue (by both fat cells and immune cells) in obesity and that it is also involved in metabolic and inflammatory processes that underlie the development of obesity-related pathologies.[14] MIF is stored in preformed pools inside immune cells, from which it is rapidly secreted when the immune cells are exposed to inflammatory and stress stimulation.[15]

Abundant evidence has demonstrated that MIF inhibits p53 and its anti-cancer functions.[16,17] Specific to this book, we know that MIF is overactive in breast cancer.[18] In fact, in an article about breast cancer, we are told that MIF inhibits induction of p53-dependent apoptosis (normal programmed cell death), increases production of vascular endothelial growth factor (VEGF), which delivers new blood vessels to growing tumors, and inhibits the antitumor immune response.[18] This should make you better appreciate what a pro-cancerous disaster it is to overeat refined sugar, flour, and oils, and to also be obese. Not surprisingly, scientists developed a drug to inhibit VEGF called Avastin and it has been used to treat breast cancer, which is typically prescribed to patients without ever letting them know that VEGF is overproduced due to a pro-inflammatory diet.

In Figure 2 in Chapter 3, recall that the dietary omega-6 (n-6) fatty acid linoleic acid (LA) is converted into arachidonic acid (AA), which then converts into prostaglandin E2 (PGE2), which stimulates aromatase and estrogen synthesis. Note that this is included in Figure 1 in this chapter. Also notice that the same PGE2 inhibits p53 to promote breast cancer expression.[12] This means that the over-consumption of omega-6 oils (corn, sunflower, safflower, cottonseed, peanut, and soybean) and grain-fed meat, fish, and chicken that are rich in omega-6 fatty acids, leads to the simultaneous inhibition of p53 and stimulation of aromatase.

As illustrated in Figure 1, a pro-inflammatory diet is also lacking in polyphenols and carotenoids, which are the anti-inflammatory pigments that give fruits and vegetables their characteristic colors. In general, the majority of polyphenols that we eat do not get absorbed into body circulation and instead exert their anti-inflammatory activity in the lumen of the intestines by DeFlaming our bacterial population. Perhaps 20-40% of polyphenols get absorbed depending on the type of vegetation you eat. In contrast, almost all ingested carotenoids are absorbed. If you would like more information on polyphenols and carotenoids, there is a chapter devoted to this topic in *The DeFlame Diet* book. With this in mind, both the absorbed polyphenols and carotenoids serve to deliver multiple anti-inflammatory benefits, including the stimulation of p53.

There are two versions of p53 in the body. The one discussed above is the health-promoting and anti-cancer p53. The second is a mutant p53 that is ineffective at inhibiting mTOR and also tends to inhibit healthy p53, which can lead to the augmentation of mTOR and related cancer expression. Approximately 50% of all cancers have a mutant p53 gene. It appears that this mutation emerges overtime as the normal cell is mutated and the cancer cell is released from apoptosis (programmed cell death) and is able to survive.[19] This suggests that the mutation is the outcome of the various pro-inflammatory factors discussed in this book. Fortunately, evidence suggests that we can reduce the damage that is delivered to p53.

If adding polyphenols to mutant p53 can reverse/disrupt the mutation, this suggests that adequate polyphenol intake, in combination with the other anti-inflammatory factors discussed in this book and *The DeFlame Diet* book, can prevent the mutation from developing in the first place. Indeed, "epidemiological studies have revealed that the risk of certain types of cancer, particularly cancers of the breast, digestive tract, skin, prostate and certain hematological malignancies, is inversely correlated with intake of polyphenols."[20] This means that as polyphenol intake increases, the likelihood of cancer expression decreases.

To understand how polyphenols and carotenoids reduce cancer expression, scientists use cancer cell models. This means these are not animal or human experiments. Scientists look at what happens to cultured cancer cells in a laboratory setting to understand treatment mechanisms. This approach is used for assessing how any possible treatment might work, be it pharmaceutical or nutritional. It should be understood that these studies are limited because the cultured cancer cells are out of the body and no longer exposed to xenoestrogens and a pro-inflammatory diet, which means that the degree of improvement that occurs in isolated cells cannot be translated to improvements that might occur in the human body that is made of many trillions of cells. From a practical perspective, this means that we should absolutely load up on polyphenol- and carotenoid-rich vegetation; it will absolutely help to varying degrees and there is no downside to worry about at all.

Multiple polyphenols have been shown to upregulate the expression of p53. Luteolin,[21] which is rich in celery and green peppers; onion polyphenols;[22] curcumin, the most potent polyphenol in turmeric;[23-25] and green tea polyphenols,[26] have all been shown to stimulate p53.

Lutein is a carotenoid found in green leafy vegetables, the most notable being cooked kale and spinach. When delivered to cultured breast tissue cells, the outcome was increased expression of p53.[27]

Glucosinolates are sulfur-containing compounds in cruciferous vegetables. They are different than botanical polyphenols or carotenoids; however, they are all anti-inflammatory phytonutrients. For our purposes of looking at p53 modulation, this distinction is not an issue. A type of glucosinolate called phenethylglucosinolate is found most concentrated in raw watercress and then broccoli. Chewing converts the phenethylglucosinolate into phenethyl isothiocyanate. The introduction of phenethyl isothiocyanate to cultured cancer cells targets the mutant p53, which allows healthy p53 to exert its tumor suppressive effect.[28,29]

Vitamin D signaling reduces the production of both PGE2 and aromatase. Vitamin D also works in concert with p53.[30] Thus, a lack of vitamin D leads to increased signaling of PGE2 and aromatase to promote cancer, and a reduction in apoptosis (normal programmed cell death), which allows cancer cells to proliferate.

You should also be aware that there is a problematic relationship between vitamin D and p53. When the mutant version of p53 emerges, it co-opts the anti-tumor effects of vitamin D, rendering it "anti-apoptotic," which means it no longer functions to promote the death of cancer cells.[31] This scenario serves as a great example of why it is foolish to focus on one intervention approach, such as vitamin D therapy, for a multi-causal and highly complex disease like cancer.

This information suggests that we need to absolutely eliminate calories from refined sugar, flour, and oils, and load up on anti-inflammatory vegetation to ensure a high intake of polyphenols, carotenoids, and other phytonutrients to eliminate the dietary drive that mutates p53. Then we are much more likely to get the anti-cancer benefit of vitamin D. For more details about vitamin D, check out *The DeFlame Diet* book.

If you carefully look at Figure 1, you will see that there are multiple ways that a pro-inflammatory diet leads to mTOR activation; this is why I stated earlier that xenoestrogens need not exist and breast cancer would still be a menace upon society. I included Figure 2 below to emphasize this fact. Notice that the xenoestrogen drive to breast cancer is absent compared to Figure 1; however, a pro-inflammatory diet by itself is capable of inhibiting p53 and stimulating mTOR and aromatase to drive breast cancer.

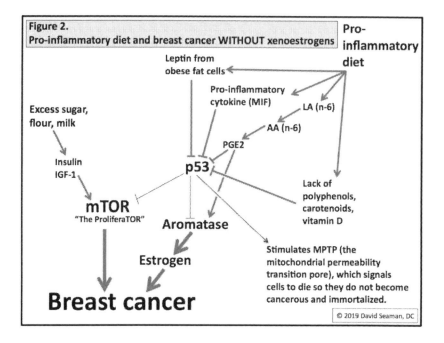

Figure 2.
Pro-inflammatory diet and breast cancer WITHOUT xenoestrogens

Envision the following common scenario and pretend we are in a xenobiotic-free world. This is because we need not be exposed to xenobiotics in order to profoundly activate mTOR. The average person spends most of their time indoors, which means most people are vitamin D deficient. You head off for a 2-week vacation at the beach. You slather up every day with sunscreen and so you block the production of anti-inflammatory vitamin D. On the way to work each day, people commonly eat a couple of donuts and drink a cup of coffee with a bunch of sugar. Later in the morning a sugary snack is consumed. For lunch, a common choice is potato chips and/or fries, a burger, and soda. For dinner people typically eat meat, fish, or chicken, French fries, bread, dessert, and no vegetables. Most people eat in this way every day, week after week, and year after year. The outcome for unlucky women is that mTOR will be progressively activated until breast cancer or some other cancer is expressed. If there is any doubt that Americans live like this, we only need to look at the most common foods consumed by Americans.

Rank	Overall, Ages 2+ yrs (Mean kcal/d; Total daily calories = 2,157)	Children and Adolescents, Ages 2-18 yrs (Mean kcal/d; Total daily calories = 2,027)	Adults and Older Adults, Ages 19+ yrs (Mean kcal/d; Total daily calories = 2,199)
1	Grain-based desserts[b] (138 kcal)	Grain-based desserts (138 kcal)	Grain-based desserts (138 kcal)
2	Yeast breads[c] (129 kcal)	Pizza (136 kcal)	Yeast breads (134 kcal)
3	Chicken and chicken mixed dishes[d] (121 kcal)	Soda/energy/sports drinks (118 kcal)	Chicken and chicken mixed dishes (123 kcal)
4	Soda/energy/sports drinks[e] (114 kcal)	Yeast breads (114 kcal)	Soda/energy/sports drinks (112 kcal)
5	Pizza (98 kcal)	Chicken and chicken mixed dishes (113 kcal)	Alcoholic beverages (106 kcal)
6	Alcoholic beverages (82 kcal)	Pasta and pasta dishes (91 kcal)	Pizza (86 kcal)
7	Pasta and pasta dishes[f] (81 kcal)	Reduced fat milk (86 kcal)	Tortillas, burritos, tacos (85 kcal)
8	Tortillas, burritos, tacos[g] (80 kcal)	Dairy desserts (76 kcal)	Pasta and pasta dishes (78 kcal)
9	Beef and beef mixed dishes[h] (64 kcal)	Potato/corn/other chips (70 kcal)	Beef and beef mixed dishes (71 kcal)
10	Dairy desserts[i] (62 kcal)	Ready-to-eat cereals (65 kcal)	Dairy desserts (58 kcal)
11	Potato/corn/other chips (56 kcal)	Tortillas, burritos, tacos (63 kcal)	Burgers (53 kcal)
12	Burgers (53 kcal)	Whole milk (60 kcal)	Regular cheese (51 kcal)
13	Reduced fat milk (51 kcal)	Candy (56 kcal)	Potato/corn/other chips (51 kcal)
14	Regular cheese (49 kcal)	Fruit drinks (55 kcal)	Sausage, franks, bacon, and ribs (49 kcal)
15	Ready-to-eat cereals (49 kcal)	Burgers (55 kcal)	Nuts/seeds and nut/seed mixed dishes (47 kcal)
16	Sausage, franks, bacon, and ribs (49 kcal)	Fried white potatoes (52 kcal)	Fried white potatoes (46 kcal)
17	Fried white potatoes (48 kcal)	Sausage, franks, bacon, and ribs (47 kcal)	Ready-to-eat cereals (44 kcal)
18	Candy (47 kcal)	Regular cheese (43 kcal)	Candy (44 kcal)
19	Nuts/seeds and nut/seed mixed dishes[j] (42 kcal)	Beef and beef mixed dishes (43 kcal)	Eggs and egg mixed dishes (42 kcal)
20	Eggs and egg mixed dishes[k] (39 kcal)	100% fruit juice, not orange/grapefruit (35 kcal)	Rice and rice mixed dishes (41 kcal)
21	Rice and rice mixed dishes[l] (36 kcal)	Eggs and egg mixed dishes (30 kcal)	Reduced fat milk (39 kcal)
22	Fruit drinks[m] (36 kcal)	Pancakes, waffles, and French toast (29 kcal)	Quickbreads (36 kcal)
23	Whole milk (33 kcal)	Crackers (28 kcal)	Other fish and fish mixed dishes[n] (30 kcal)
24	Quickbreads[o] (32 kcal)	Nuts/seeds and nut/seed mixed dishes (27 kcal)	Fruit drinks (29 kcal)
25	Cold cuts (27 kcal)	Cold cuts (24 kcal)	Salad dressing (29 kcal)

TABLE 2 2. Top 25 Sources of Calories Among Americans Ages 2 Years and Older, NHANES 2005-2006[a]

The above image is part of Table 2-2, which lists the 25 most commonly eaten food by Americans aged 2 and older. It came from Dietary Guidelines for Americans 2010, which was published by the United States Department of Agriculture (USDA). The full document is free and can be acquired by doing an internet search of the title. Notice that the primary calories consumed by all age groups are refined sugar, flour, oils, milk, meat, chicken, and cheese. No vegetables or fruit make the top 25 most commonly consumed foods in any category. Clearly, this lifestyle represents a "pursuit" of breast cancer and other cancers, and xenoestrogens need not be present for cancer to emerge. And if we do add xenoestrogens into the mix, which does impact most of us, it just adds more fuel to the inhibition of p53 and stimulation of mTOR and aromatase, and the aggressive march toward cancer.

Cigarette smoking

Multiple xenobiotic agents are found in cigarettes. There are approximately 70 carcinogenic materials out of the total 7,000 chemicals in cigarettes.[32] The most notable and studied carcinogens include polycyclic aromatic hydrocarbons and tobacco-specific nitrosamines.[32] The xenobiotics in cigarettes promote breast cancer by several mechanisms, which are beyond the scope of this book. One of the ways that was described in detail earlier is via the activation of NF-kB.[32]

Not surprisingly, the best option for smokers is to quit. The problem is that quitting is difficult. If you cannot quit, try to limit smoking to an absolute minimum. Additionally, it has been shown that aerobic exercise seems to reduce the lung injury associated with smoking.[33] This may translate into reduced systemic inflammation, which would be of benefit to breast health. There is also evidence from animal models that supplementation with curcumin from turmeric reduces the pro-inflammatory damage induced by smoking.[34]

References

1. https://www.cdc.gov/biomonitoring/Phthalates_FactSheet.html
2. Godet I, Gllkes DM. BRCA1 and BRCA2 mutations and treatment strategies for breast cancer. Integr Cancer Sci Ther. 2017;4: 10.15761/ICST.1000228.
3. Olson AC, Link JS, Waisman JR, Kupiec TC. Breast cancer patients unknowingly dosing themselves with estrogen by using topic moisturizers. J Clin Oncol. 2009;27:e103-104.
4. Donovan M, Tiwary CM, Axelrod D, et al. Personal care products that contain estrogens or xenoestrogens may increase breast cancer risk. Med Hypoth. 2007;68:756-66.
5. Hutz RJ, Carvan MJ, Larson JK, et al. Familiar and novel reproductive endocrine disruptors: xenoestrogens, dioxins, and nanoparticles. Curr Trends Endocrinol. 2014;7:111-122.
6. Goodson WH, Luciani MG, Sayeed SA, et al. Activation of the mTOR pathway by low levels of xenoestrogens in breast epithelial cells from high-risk women. Carcinogenesis. 2011;32:1724-33.

7. Dairkee SH, Luciani-Torres MG, Moore DH, Goodson WH. Bisphenol-A-induced inactivation of the p53 axis underlying deregulation of proliferation kinetics, and cell death in non-malignant human breast epithelial cells. Carcinogenesis. 2013;34:703-12.

8. Li J, Kim SG, Blenis J. Rapamycin: one drug, many effects. Cell Metab. 2014;19:373-79.

9. Yoon MS. mTOR as a key regulator in maintaining skeletal muscle mass. Front Physiol. 2017;8:788.

10. Feng Z, Zhang H, Levine AJ, Jin S. The coordinate regulation of the p53 and mTOR pathways in cells. Proc Natl Acad Sci USA. 2005;102:8204-209.

11. Vaseva AV, Moll UM. The mitochondrial p53 pathway. Biochim Biophys Acta. 1787:414-20.

12. Wang X, Docanto MM, Sasano H, et al. Prostaglandin E2 inhibits p53 in human breast adipose stromal cells: a novel mechanism for the regulation of aromatase in obesity and breast cancer. Cancer Res. 2015;75:645-55.

13. Finucane OM, Reynolds CM, McGillicuddy FC, Roche HM. Insights into the role of macrophage migration inhibitory factor in obesity and insulin resistance. Proc Nutr Soc. 2012;71:622-33.

14. Morrison MC, Kleemann R. Role of macrophage migration inhibitory factor in obesity, insulin resistance, type 2 diabetes, and associated co-morbidities: a comprehensive review of human and rodent studies. Front Immunol. 2015;6:308.

15. Heinrichs D, Berres ML, Coeuru M, et al. Protective role of macrophage migration inhibitory factor in nonalcoholic steatohepatitis. FASEB J. 2014;28:5136-47.

16. Hudson JD, Shoaibi MA, Maestro R, et al. A proinflammatory cytokine inhibits p53 tumor suppressor activity. J Exp Med. 1999;190:1375-82.

17. Conroy H, Mawhinney L, Donnelly SC. Inflammation and cancer: macrophage migration inhibitory factor (MIF)—the potential missing link. Q J Med. 2010;103:831-36

18. Richard V, Kindt N, Saussez S. Macrophage migration inhibitory factor involvement in breast cancer (review). Int J Oncol. 2015;47:1627-33.

19. Rivlin N, Brosh R, Oren M, Rotter V. Mutations in the p53 tumor suppressor gene: important milestones at the various steps of tumorigenesis. Genes Cancer. 2011;2:466-74.

20. Liu R, Ji P, Liu B, et al. Apigenin enhances the cisplatin cytotoxic effect through p53-modulated apoptosis. Oncol Lett. 2017;13:1024-30.

21. Lin Y, Shi R, Wang X, Shen HM. Luteolin, a flavonoid with potentials for cancer prevention and therapy. Curr Cancer Drug Targets. 2008;8:634-46.

22. Lee WS, Yi SM, Yun JW, et al. Polyphenols isolated from Allium cep L. induces apoptosis by induction of p53 and suppression of Bcl-2 through inhibiting PI3K/Akt signaling pathway in AGS human cancer cells. J Cancer Prev. 2014;19:14-22.

23. Talib WH, Al-hadid SA, Ali MB, et al. Role of curcumin in regulating p53 in breast cancer: an overview of the mechanism of action. Breast Cancer. 2018;10:207-17.

24. He ZY, Shi CB, Wen H, et al. Upregulation of p53 expression in patients with colorectal cancer by administration of curcumin. Cancer Invest. 2011;29:208-13.

25. Hallman K, Aleck K, Dwyer B, et al. The effects of turmeric (curcumin) on tumor suppressor protein (p53) and estrogen receptor (ER) in breast cancer cells. Breast Cancer. 2017;9:153-61.

26. Gupta K, Thakur VS, Bhaskaran N, et al. Green tea polyphenols induce p53-dependent and p53-independent apoptosis in prostate cancer cells through two distinct mechanisms. PLoS ONE. 2012;7:e52572.

27. Chew BP, Park JS. Carotenoid action on the immune response. J Nutr. 2004;134:257S-261S.

28. Aggarwal M, Saxena R, Sinclair E, et al. Reactivation of mutant p53 by a dietary-related compound phenethyl isothiocyanate inhibits tumor growth. Cell Death Differ. 2016;23:1615-27.

29. Gupta P, Wright SE, Kim SH Srivistava SK. Phenethyl isothiocyanate: a comprehensive review of anti-cancer mechanisms. Biochem Biophys Acta. 2014;1846:405-24

30. Patel JB, Pate KD, Patel SR et al. Recent candidate molecular markers: vitamin D signaling and apoptosis specific regulator of p53 (ASPP) in breast cancer. Asian Pacific J Cancer Prev. 2012;13:1727-35.

31. Stambolsky P, Tabach Y, Fontemaggi G, et al. Modulation of the vitamin D response by cancer associated mutant p53. Cancer Cell. 2010;17:273-85.

32. Kispert S, McHowat J. Recent insights into cigarette smoking as a lifestyle risk factor for breast cancer. Breast Cancer. 2017;9:127-32.

33. Toledo AC, Magalhaes RM, Hizume DC, et al. Aerobic exercise attenuates pulmonary injury induced by exposure to cigarette smoke. Eur Respir J. 2012;39:254-64.

34. Lian Z, Wu R, Xie W, et al. Curcumin reverses tobacco smoke-induced epithelial-mesenchymal transition by suppressing the MAPK pathway in the lungs of mice. Mol Med Rep. 2018;17:2019-25.

Chapter 7
EGF, EGFR and HER2 in breast cancer

In the previous chapters, I discussed how two growth factors (VEGF and IGF-1) promote breast cancer. This chapter is specifically about another growth factor called epidermal growth factor (EGF). All growth factors bind to receptors, which then initiates cell growth. In the case of EGF, it can bind to two receptors; one is called epidermal growth factor receptor (EGFR) or human epidermal growth factor receptor 1 (HER1), and the second is human epidermal growth factor receptor 2 (HER2), the outcome of which is cell growth.

The activity of EGF is needed for wound healing, which involves cellular growth and tissue repair. The problem is when EGF activity is up-regulated and promotes uncontrolled cell growth, which is the case with breast cancer. An over expression of both EGF receptors (HER1 and HER2) is associated with larger tumor size, enhanced disease expression, and poorer clinical outcomes. An over expression of HER1 occurs in about 15-30% of breast cancers and HER2 over expression is observed in 20-30% of cases.[1]

Testing for HER2 is most common in the clinical setting and is typically reserved for more invasive cancer cases. Several medications are available for HER2-positive patients, such as lapatinib (Tykerb), neratinib (Nerlynx), pertuzumab (Perjeta), trastuzumab (Herceptin), and others.

From the perspective of nutrition, we know that leptin increases HER2 levels in breast cancer cells.[2] Leptin is over-produced by obese fat cells, a topic that will be discussed in the next chapter. Leptin production by fat cells will normalize by dietary caloric restriction that reduces obesity. Similarly, caloric restriction has been shown to reduce HER1 activity and related IGF-1 activity.[3] In other words, it is very important to achieve a normal body weight and related markers of inflammation, the theme of *The DeFlame Diet*, which can help to promote a normal expression of growth factors related to cancer expression. Consider the following case history.

A 66-year old woman was diagnosed with recurrent breast cancer and was scheduled for surgery in three weeks.[4] The pre-surgical biopsy was both estrogen receptor positive and also positive for HER2. Immediately upon receiving the diagnosis, the woman began a strict ketogenic diet and also supplemented with 10,000 IU of vitamin D3. After the tumor was removed, it was tested again and found to be no longer positive for HER2, which means nutrition has the power to modify cancer expression. While this is only a single case history, it should not stop one from being very pro-active with *The DeFlame Diet*.

References
1. Hsu JL, Hung MC. The role of HER2, EGFR, and other receptor kinases in breast cancer. Cancer Metastasis Rev. 2016;35:575-588.
2. Giordano C, Vizza D, Panza S, et al. Leptin increases HER2 protein levels through a STAT3-mediated up-regulation of Hsp90 in breast cancer cells. Mol Oncol. 2013;7:379-91.
3. Moore T, Checkley LA, DiGiovanni J. Dietary energy balance modulation of epithelial carcinogenesis: a role for IGF-1 receptor signaling and crosstalk. Ann NY Acad Sci.
4. Branca JJ, Pacini S, Ruggiero M. Effects of pre-surgical vitamin D supplementation and ketogenic diet in a patient with recurrent breast cancer. Anticancer Res. 2015;35:5525-32.

Chapter 8
Obesity and breast cancer

People still misunderstand obesity to be merely a condition of excess calorie storage. In fact, obesity is a chronic inflammatory state that promotes all chronic diseases, including breast cancer. Multiple studies have found that obese women with breast cancers have consistently poorer prognosis, larger tumors and lymph node metastasis.[1] Studies indicate that obesity is associated with increased risk of more aggressive breast cancer. Obese women are likely to have metastatic breast cancer when they are first diagnosed and to have a poor prognosis regardless of their menopausal status.[2]

With the above in mind, there is a strong relationship between obesity in postmenopausal women and breast cancer development, but a less consistent relationship to obesity in premenopausal women.[1] My suspicion is this has to do with the chronic nature of the obesity state.

First, it is important to understand that, as we age, we naturally "flame up"; this is the case for everyone. Dying of old age is the ultimate inflammatory event – no specific chronic disease is required. We cannot live forever, even if we are physically active, lean, fit, or free of disease.

Scientists use the term "inflammaging" to describe the inflammatory changes associated with the normal aging process. The goal should be to *not* exaggerate and accelerate the inflammaging process, which is why obesity is such a problem. Obesity is always associated with an uptick in inflammation; however, this is less severe when we are young and becomes progressively more severe as we inflammage. Additionally, in most cases, older obese individuals have been obese for many decades, which means that they have lived with the chronic inflammatory state of obesity for an extended number of years while they were simultaneously inflammaging.

Three cancers are often considered to be obesity-related cancers, including cancers of breast, prostate, and colon.[3] Obviously, prostate is unique to males, while breast is most common in female; however, the incidence of breast cancer in males is rising. Colon cancer, of course, emerges in both men and women.

What is it about obesity that is promotional for cancer? Part of the problem is elevated blood glucose levels and related problems, which will be the focus of the next chapter. In the present chapter, we are going to focus on pro-inflammatory and pro-cancerous biochemistry that exists in body fat that serves to "flame up" the entire body. Body fat is made up of two primary cell types, those being fat cells and immune cells, which together create the adipose organ.

Fat cells (adipocytes)
Fat cells, also called adipocytes, produce three important hormones, including adiponectin, leptin, and visfatin. A fourth hormone called resistin is released by macrophages (a white blood cell) associated with obese fat cells. Each has been studied in the context of breast cancer expression, as well as other obesity related diseases, the most notable being diabetes and heart disease. Because three of these hormones are secreted by adipocytes, they are collectively referred to as adipokines or adipocytokines. Each will be discussed below.

Adiponectin
Adiponectin production levels by fat cells are directly related to adiposity, which means the degree of body fatness. Fat cells can either be lean, overweight, or obese, or in transition among one of these three states. Lean fat cells produce proper amounts of adiponectin, which is then released into body circulation to deliver multiple anti-inflammatory functions. As body fatness increases, there is a commensurate reduction in adiponectin production, and therefore, less adiponectin in circulation and less anti-inflammatory activity throughout the body. Here is a list of the anti-inflammatory effects of adiponectin that are lost as one progresses toward the chronic inflammatory state of obesity:[4]

Skeletal muscle: increases fat burning (properly called fat oxidation for energy production), increases skeletal muscle response to insulin

Liver: reduces inflammation, reduces fibrosis, reduces fat infiltration, reduces the production of glucose

Fat cells: increases glucose uptake, which helps to maintain normal blood glucose levels

Brain: increases energy expenditure, reduces body weight

Macrophages (a specific immune cell): reduces foam cell formation, which prevents vascular disease called atherosclerosis

Heart: helps to maintain vascular regulation to prevent ischemic injury, which means injury due to reduced blood flow

Endothelial cells (the cells that line all blood vessel walls, which is 60-100 thousand miles of blood vessels inside the human body): increases vasodilation (vessel relaxation to improve blood supply to vital organs), reduces adhesion molecules (substances the causes immune cells to stick to each other and to vessel walls)

Smooth muscle (the muscles in blood vessel walls that contract/relax and promote atherosclerosis when chronic inflammation is present): reduces their proliferation and migration, which means adiponectin prevents atherosclerosis

Pancreas: protects insulin-producing cells from injury by pro-inflammatory cytokines

In the context of breast cancer specifically, here is what adiponectin does. First, adiponectin reduces aromatase activity, which is responsible for the excess production of estrogen that promotes breast cancer. Second, adiponectin reduces the expression of estrogen receptors on breast cancer cells. Third, adiponectin represses cancer proliferation in cell studies that examined both estrogen-receptor positive and negative breast cancer.[5]

It is important to remember that adiponectin is only released in proper amounts by non-obese and therefore, non-inflamed fat cells. And because fat cell-derived adiponectin improves the function of multiple organs and even prevents breast cancer, you can see why it is ridiculous to view fat cells as just a place where excess calories are stored. If your fat cells are lean, they will help DeFlame your entire body…quite amazing.

However, if our fat mass increases, particularly our abdominal fat mass, all of these beneficial functions of adiponectin are lost to varying degrees, and no drug or nutritional supplement can correct these multiple deficits. Even if one is not worried about cancer, it is quite obvious why we want to be lean and maintain adequate adiponectin production, as it is involved with so many vital body functions.

Two final points about adiponectin for you to think about. First, adiponectin levels in the blood supply are supposed to be 1000-fold higher compared to many pro-inflammatory growth factors and cytokines,[6] which is likely how it is able to participate in so many important anti-inflammatory functions. Second, adiponectin also appears to be a systemic (full body/most cells) down-regulator of NF-kB.[6] The only way to maintain or restore normal adiponectin levels is to achieve a normal lean body weight. At the present time, in 2019, approximately 70% of the adult population is overweight or obese.

Leptin

Leptin is the other hormone produced exclusively by fat cells (adipocytes). In contrast to adiponectin, which is reduced by obesity, leptin release is increased, such that obese people are described to have hyperleptinemia, which means abnormally elevated blood levels of leptin. What does this mean for breast cancer risk or a case of active breast cancer?

Breast cancer cells express leptin receptors. The reason for this is because cancer cells benefit from high levels of leptin. Leptin functions to both enhance the signaling pathways involved in tumor proliferation and simultaneously, it down regulates the normal apoptosis (cell death) process, allowing potentially cancerous cells that should be killed to escape and proliferate.[5] For example, a tumor suppressor gene, called p53, functions to stop the formation of tumors, which was discussed and illustrated in Chapter 6. As described in Chapter 5 and 6, elevated levels of leptin inhibit p53,[5] which is needed to generate the mitochondrial permeability transition pore (MPTP), which prevents cells from becoming cancerous.[7] Leptin also stimulates aromatase activity, which as described earlier, leads to an over-production of estrogen that promotes breast cancer. Leptin also stimulates angiogenesis (new blood vessel growth),[5] which is required for tumors to grow. As described in the last chapter, leptin also stimulates HER2 production in breast cancer cells.

Visfatin

The majority of visfatin production appears to come from visceral adipose tissue, although subcutaneous adipose tissue is also a producer. Visceral fat, as the name indicates, is the fat that accumulates around visceral organs, rather than subcutaneous, which is obviously the fat that accumulates beneath the skin. As people overeat, both visceral and subcutaneous fat deposits increase. Not surprisingly, circulating levels of visfatin increase with obesity.[8] This is a problem for women at risk for breast cancer. Visfatin has been identified as a promoter of breast cancer.[9-11]

Resistin

Resistin was named because it was first correlated to insulin resistance. It was discovered around the year 2000 and was first found to be released by adipocytes in rodents. However, in humans, it is predominantly secreted by a type of pro-inflammatory white blood cell called an M1 macrophage, which is found in obese adipose tissue.[12] Elevated circulating levels of resistin correlate to body fat accumulation, which is likely why it is still commonly referred to as an adipokine. In short, elevated levels of resistin are significantly associated with breast cancer expression.[13] In addition to promoting insulin resistance, resistin also functions as an activator of NF-kB,[14] which was described earlier as a key signaling molecule in driving the chronic inflammatory state.

The only way to normalize adiponectin, leptin, visfatin, and resistin levels to reduce chronic inflammation, is to normalize your body weight. No drug or nutritional supplement can do it for us.

Body fat immune cells

One of the first studies that identified immune cells in adipose tissue was published in 2003.[15] This is an extremely new finding in science and has changed the way we look at body fatness. Historically, overweight or obese individuals were merely viewed as carriers of excess stored calories. Now we know that adipose tissue is an organ, comprised of two major cell types, those being adipocytes and immune cells, each of which produces numerous chemicals that influence local adipose tissue physiology and systemic (full body) physiology.

When we are young and lean, which historically was the case for almost all adolescents, both fat and immune cells release anti-inflammatory chemicals. As we age and become stressed out and sedentary overeaters, we start to pack on the fat pounds and this causes both fat and immune cells to release pro-inflammatory chemicals that participate in promoting all of the well-known chronic diseases, such as diabetes, osteoarthritis, heart disease, and cancer.[16] The transformation of lean adipose tissue that contains healthy anti-inflammatory fat cells and immune cells, to obese adipose tissue with pro-inflammatory fat cells and immune cells is called "adipose tissue remodeling."[17]

It is important to understand that the immune cell profile in obese remodeled adipose tissue resembles that of an infection or autoimmune disease. I personally think we should view obesity as a state of being "infected" by excess calories, to which the immune system responds accordingly by releasing a host of pro-inflammatory chemicals, which would otherwise be released only if there is an actual microbial or viral infection. Scientists, in the laboratory setting, have demonstrated that this sentiment is true.

A point of clarification before continuing…it is a mistake to think that our stored fat comes mostly from the fat we eat. In fact, the majority of calories we eat come from refined sugar and flour, which makes up approximately 40% of all the calories Americans consume. The excess sugar/flour calories we eat is converted into *saturated* fat and stored in adipocytes. For more information about saturated fat, unsaturated fat, trans fat, and cholesterol, check out *The DeFlame Diet* book that contains 60 pages about these topics.

There are two key immune-activating events that occur as adipocytes fill up with fat. One involves a reduction in oxygen levels within the expanding adipose tissue mass, referred to as hypoxia. The local hypoxia cause adipocytes to release chemotactic agents, which attract immune cells to enter the hypoxic fat mass.[17,18] As obese fat cells age, they become necrotic and release their abundance of saturated fatty acids. It turns out that the receptor for microbial antigens (infective proteins) on immune cells, called a Toll-like receptor-4 (TLR4), also responds to the saturated fatty acids that are released by necrotic fat cells.[17] Additionally, it appears that resistin, which was described earlier, can also activate TLR4.[14] This means that non-microbial factors are capable of activating the immune system to behave like a chronic low-grade infection is present – in the case of the majority of Americans, we become chronically "infected," not by viruses or bacteria, but by excess calories from sugar, flour, and refined oils.

One of the immune cells found in obese adipose tissue is called a macrophage, whose function is to engulf microbes; however, there are no microbes in body fat. The macrophages show up in abundance to engulf the fat-laden and necrotic adipocytes, as if it they were microbes. In fact, 90% of the macrophages that enter obese adipose tissue are there to deal with necrotic fat cells.[19]

Scientists have examined the structural relationship between necrotic fat cells and macrophages, which is referred to as a crown-like structure.[19] Figure 1, which is nicely colorized in the Kindle version of this book, illustrates the difference in cell types that make up lean adipose tissue and obese adipose tissue.[20-23] Notice how fat cells swell in size as they take in calories and become obese. Also notice how the immune cell population completely changes when lean fat cells are transformed into obese fat cells, and M1 macrophages encircle the necrotic fat cell to create what looks like a crown.

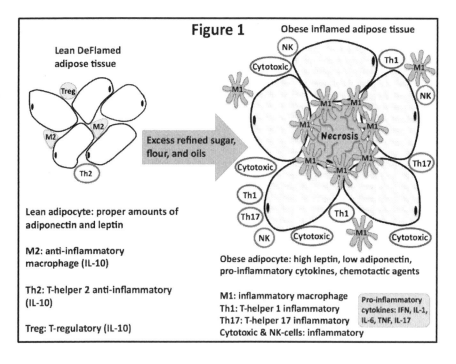

Recall from above that lean adipocytes produce the adiponectin that circulates at 1000xs the level of pro-inflammatory growth factors and cytokines (IL-1, IL-6, IL-17, TNF, etc.). Lean adipocytes progressively lose the ability to produce adiponectin as they become increasingly more obese, which eventually leads to a depressed level of adiponectin in body circulation, which is highly inflammatory. Simultaneously, obese adipocytes do not lose their ability to release leptin; in fact, leptin levels in circulation significantly increase, which is highly pro-inflammatory as discussed earlier in this chapter.

Notice also in Figure 1 that lean adipose tissue contains at least three different anti-inflammatory immune cells, all of which release an extremely important anti-inflammatory cytokine called interleukin-10 (IL-10). The anti-inflammatory macrophage is designated as M2. The other two cells are anti-inflammatory T lymphocytes. One is called a T-helper 2 cell (Th2). The second is a T-regulatory cell (Treg), which releases anti-inflammatory IL-10 and also functions to promote self-tolerance, which means they prevent autoimmune disease expression. Clearly, we all need to have lean anti-inflammatory adipose tissue. Unfortunately, during the obesity process, anti-inflammatory fat cells and immune cells are replaced by those that are pro-inflammatory and capable of perpetually releasing pro-inflammatory chemistry 24 hours per day, which is augmented whenever excess calories are consumed.

The obese adipose tissue illustrated in Figure 1 should scare you…it scares me for sure. Life is difficult enough on so many levels for the average person that no one should self-impose an additional layer of misery on themselves by moving through life with necrotic fat cells in their bodies.

Th1 cells (T-helper 1 cells) typically participate in autoimmune disease expression, rheumatoid arthritis and psoriasis being the most well-known. Th1 cells release a cytokine called interferon (IFN) which causes neighboring immune cells, particularly M1 macrophages to release their pro-inflammatory cytokines (IL-1, IL-6, TNF). When IFN was used to treat patients with chronic active hepatitis C, 40% of subjects developed full-blown major depression.[24]

Th17 (T-helper 17 cells) were discovered more recently compared to Th1 and Th2 cells. They were named based on their release of interleukin-17 (IL-17), another pro-inflammatory cytokine. The main role of IL-17 in humans is to combat bacterial and fungal infections,[25] however, Th-17 cells rapidly accumulate in obese adipose tissue,[22] which, as stated above, is "infected" with excess calories and not microorganisms. IL-17 production is involved in the expression of multiple diseases, including breast cancer.[22] Here is an additional consideration to help motivate you to DeFlame…it turns out that elevated levels of IL-17 in a pregnant woman will bathe the brain of the developing fetus for 9 months, rendering it more vulnerable to expressing autism.[26]

Cytotoxic T-cells and natural killer (NK) cells typically show up to release pro-inflammatory cytokines to combat cancer and viral infections. This information should again alert you to the fact that the human body perceives obesity as a biochemical state that resembles an autoimmune disease, an infection, and/or cancer. No one should be surprised why obese individuals are far more likely to be fatigued, lethargic, depressed, and in physical pain compared to their lean counterparts.

The pro-inflammatory transformation illustrated in Figure 1 occurs anywhere that obese fat cells become hypoxic and necrotic, and this includes breast tissue. Indeed, fat cells in the breast absolutely "flame up" during the obesity state, become necrotic, and then participate in the local inflammation that promotes breast cancer expression.[27-29] In other words, the way to view this necrotic process is to conceptualize that it exists in breast tissue long before breast cancer becomes established.

Unfortunately, the average American (70% of us) is either overweight or obese. This means that adipose tissue is remodeled to varying degrees in all of these individuals and resembles, to varying degrees, the pro-inflammatory adipose tissue image in Figure 1. Clearly, women should not pursue a lifestyle that leads to the development of necrotic fat cell accumulation in breast tissue, which represents both a pre-cancerous and cancerous state. This means that the entire family should engage in the DeFlaming process, which starts when kids are young. Now, more than any time in history, we are witnessing a shocking increase in childhood obesity, which sets the stage for the development of multiple chronic diseases. In the case of young girls, the over-consumption of refined sugar, flour, and oil calories promotes obesity and creates a biochemical environment for breast tissue to program and facilitate the expression of breast cancer.

Steps to take to get obesity under control
Many people do not realize how overweight or obese they actually are. My suggestion is to do an internet search for BMI NIH, which will take you the NIH's website where you can insert your height and weight. Your goal is to be below 25. Next, you want to check your waist/hip ratio and make sure, as a woman, yours is below .8. My suggestion is to get *The DeFlame Diet* book and carefully track all your inflammatory markers and get them all into normal levels.

You should also read *Weight Loss Secrets You Need To Know*, which outlines how to mentally get control of your eating, which is commonly called mindfulness. All the key barriers and challenges to effective weight management are presented in a fashion that will allow you to become the master of your eating environment. This book is only $.99 cents for the Kindle version and $12.95 for the paperback.

It is not just important to control your caloric intake in general, and to specifically eliminate calories from refined sugar, flour, and oil. You also need to dramatically increase your consumption of vegetation, which are loaded with vitamins, minerals, and anti-inflammatory pigments called polyphenols/carotenoids (see the chapter on polyphenols/carotenoids in *The DeFlame Diet* book). Specific to breast cancer, a recent animal model demonstrated that dietary polyphenols were able to suppress elevated levels of pro-inflammatory chemicals in the mammary gland of obese mice and also down-regulate the expression of aromatase.[30]

Not surprisingly, exercise is very important for weight management; however, there is a better way to view exercise…it is an extremely anti-inflammatory activity so long as you exercise within your

64

individual tolerance zone. Too little exercise is not enough for DeFlaming purposes, and too much can be pro-inflammatory. Consider, for example, that exercise training reduces the expression of TLR4 (the Toll-like receptor described above) on immune cells, which helps to down-regulate the inflammatory state.[31] Exercise also reduces oxidative stress (excess free radical production) and improves mitochondrial function so that fats and ketones can be readily used as energy.[31] Exercise also increases the body's production of IL-10, the powerful anti-inflammatory cytokine described earlier, and reduces immune cell production of TNF.[31] There is also evidence from an obese animal model that exercise can promote the switch from a pro-inflammatory M1 macrophage population to the anti-inflammatory M2 macrophage in adipose tissue.[32] So, clearly, we should all be engaged in exercise.

References
1. Xu YXZ, Mishra S. Obesity-linked cancers: current knowledge, challenges and limitations in mechanistic studies and rodent models. Cancers. 2018. Dec 18;10(12). pii: E523. doi: 10.3390/cancers10120523.
2. Assiri AD, Kamel HF, Hassanien MF. Resistin, visfatin, adiponectin, and leptin: risk of breast cancer in pre- and postmenopausal Saudi females and their possible diagnostic and predictive implications as novel biomarkers. Diseases Markers. 2015;
3. Murthy NS, Mukherjee S, Ray G, Ray A. Dietary factors and cancer chemoprevention: an overview of obesity-related malignancies. J Postgrad Med. 2009;55:45-54.
4. Xu A, Wang Y, Lam KS. Adiponectin. In: Fantuzzi G, Mazzone T, Eds. Adipose tissue and adipokines in health and disease. Totowa, NJ: Human Press; 2007: p.47-59.
5. Jarde T, Perrier S, Vasson MP, Caldefie-Chezet F. Molecular mechanisms of leptin and adiponectin. Eur J Cancer. 2011;47:33-43.
6. Ouchi N, Walsh K. A novel role for adiponectin in the regulation of inflammation. Arterioscler Thromb Vasc Biol. 2008;28:1219-21.
7. Vaseva AV, Moll UM. The mitochondrial p53 pathway. Biochim Biophys Acta. 2009;1787:414-20.
8. Sethi JK, Vidal-Puig A. Visfatin: the missing link between intra-abdominal obesity and diabetes? Trends Mol Med. 2005;11:344-47.
9. Lee YC, Yang YH, Su JH, et al. High visfatin expression in breast cancer tissue is associated with poor survival. Cancer Epidemiol Biomarkers Prev. 2011;20:1892-901.
10. Park HJ, Kim SR, Kim SS, et al. Visfatin promotes cell and tumor growth by upregulating Notch1 in breast cancer. Oncotarget. 2014;5:5087-99.

11. Hung AC, Lo S, Hou MF, et al. Extracellular visfatin-promoted malignant behavior in breast cancer is mediated through c-Abl and STAT3 activation. 2016;22:4478-90.

12. Schwartz DR, Lazar MA. Human resistin: found in translation from mouse to man. Trends Endocrinol Metab. 2011;22:259-65.

13. Gui Y, Pan Q, Chen X, et al. The association between obesity related adipokines and risk of breast cancer: a meta-analysis. Oncotarget. 2017;8:75389-99.

14. Codoner-Franch P, Alonso-Iglesias E. Resistin: insulin resistance to malignancy. Clin Chim Acta. 2015;438:46-54.

15. Weisberg SP, McCann D, Desai M, et al. Obesity is associated with macrophage accumulation in adipose tissue. J Clin Invest. 2003;112:1796-1808.

16. Seaman DR. Body mass index and musculoskeletal pain: is there a connection? Chiro Man Ther. 2013;21:15.

17. Sun K, Kusminski CM, Scherer PE. Adipose tissue remodeling and obesity. J Clin Invest. 2011;121:2094-2101.

18. Ferrante AW. The immune cells in adipose tissue. Diabetes Obes Meta. 2013;15:34-38.

19. Murano I, Barbatelli G, Parisani V, et al. Dead adipocytes, detected as crown-like structures, are prevalent in visceral fat depots of genetically obese mice. J Lipid Res. 2008;49:1562-68.

20. Harford KA, Reynolds CM, McGillicuddy FC, Roche HM. Fats, inflammation and insulin resistance: insights to the role of macrophage and T-cell accumulation. In adipose tissue. Proc Nutr Soc. 2011;70:408-17.

21. Cautivo KM, Molofsky AB. Regulation of metabolic health and adipose tissue function by group 2 innate lymphoid cells. Eur J Immunol. 2016;46:1315-25.

22. Chehimi M, Vidal H, Eljaafari A. Pathogenic role of IL-17-producing immune cells in obesity, and related inflammatory disease. J Clin Med. 2017;6:68.

23. Reilly SM, Saltiel AR. Adapting to obesity with adipose tissue inflammation. Nat Rev Endocrinol. 2017;13:633-43.

24. Bonaccorso S, Meltzer H, Maees M. Psychological and behavioral effects of interferons. Curr Opin Psychiatry. 2000;13:673-677.

25. Yang B, Kang H, Fung A, et al. The role of interleukin-17 in tumour proliferation, angiogenesis, and metastasis. Mediators Inflamm. 2014:623759.

26. Estes ML, McAllister AK. Maternal Th17 cells take a toll on baby's brain. Science. 2016;351:919-20.

27. Vaysse C, Lomo J, Garred O, et al. Inflammation of mammary adipose tissue occurs in overweight and obese patients exhibiting early-stage breast cancer. NPJ Breast Cancer. 2017;3:19.

28. Morris PG, Hudis CA, Giri D, et al. Inflammation and increased aromatase expression occur in the breast tissue of obese women with breast cancer. Cancer Prev Res. 2011;4:1021-29.

29. Jee J, Hong BS, Ryu HS, et al. Transition into inflammatory cancer-associated adipocytes in breast cancer microenvironment requires microRNA regulatory mechanism. PLoS ONE. 2017;12(3): e0174126.

30. Subbaramaiah K, Sue E, Bhardwaj P, et al. Dietary polyphenols suppress elevated levels of proinflammatory mediators and aromatase in the mammary gland of obese mice. Cancer Pre Res. 2013;6:886-97.

31. Kruger K. Inflammation during obesity – pathophysiological concepts and effects of physical activity. Dtsch Z Sportmed. 2017;68:163-69.

32. Kawanishi N, Yano H, Yokogawa Y, Suzuki K. Exercise training inhibits inflammation in adipose tissue via both suppression of macrophage infiltration and acceleration of phenotypic switching from M1 to M2 macrophages in high-fat-diet-induced obese mice. Exerc Immunol Rev. 2010;16:105-18.

Chapter 9
Metabolic syndrome and breast cancer

Metabolic syndrome drives cancer in many ways, however, hyperglycemia is the most obvious issue. As described in Chapter 5, the cancer cells of tumors have been described to be "addicted to blood sugar." The reason for this is because tumors derive their energy predominantly from glycolysis, which can only utilize sugar for energy production. Recall from Chapter 5 that mitochondria, which burn sugar, ketones, and fat, are no longer operational in immortalized tumor cells. In other words, the mitochondria in tumor cells are no longer making energy and also unable to initiate the cell death signaling that is required to prevent cells from transforming into cancer cells. This allows cancer cells to live on in an aggressive fashion, in which they are fully dependent on a constant supply of glucose for their survival. As also mentioned and illustrated in Figure 1 in Chapter 6, high glucose levels are associated with elevated levels of insulin and IGF-1, which activates mTOR to stimulate the proliferation of cancer cells.

It is impossible to have the metabolic syndrome if waist/hip ratio is less than .8 for females and .95 for males, fasting glucose is below 100 mg/dL, and 2-hour postprandial glucose is well below 140 mg/dL. Everyone should make it their goal to achieve and maintain these values, as well as the other markers of inflammation outlined in *The DeFlame Diet* book.

Table 1 outlines the values for the various markers that establish the criteria for the pro-inflammatory metabolic syndrome. Three of the five markers must be present in order to make the diagnosis.

Table 1 - Metabolic syndrome markers

Metabolic syndrome	Abnormal value	Date	Date	Date	Date
1. Fasting blood glucose	≥ 100 mg/dL				

2. Fasting triglycerides	≥ 150 mg/dL				
3. Fasting HDL cholesterol	< 50 for women; < 40 men				
4. Blood pressure	≥ 130/85				
5. Waist circumference	> 35" women; > 40" men				

If you have the metabolic syndrome, the first goal is to reduce the markers below the cutoff points for the metabolic syndrome. Next you must set your sights on reaching the most deflamed values for these markers. The goal for fasting glucose should be less than 80 mg/dL; the goal for fasting triglycerides is less than 90 mg/dl; fasting HDL should be 10 or more above the cutoffs; blood pressure should be below 120/80; and unless one has a large frame, the waist circumference goal for women should be 28" or less and men should be 33" or less. If one achieves these values, there will be very little metabolic drive to promote and feed cancer. For some it is easy to achieve these ideal levels; for others it takes a bit of effort. If the latter applies to you, just be patient and committed.

My 2018 book, *Weight Loss Secrets You Need To Know*, can be very helpful for those who struggle to achieve normal markers of inflammation. This book outlines the many physiological, psychological, and primordial barriers we must overcome to achieve and maintain normal body weight. The last thing you want to do is get involved in an ideological quagmire about whether you should adopt vegan (plant-based), omnivore, carnivore, ketogenic, or paleolithic diet. People can achieve normal markers of inflammation with any of these approaches. It is also possible to become obese with any of these approaches if one eats too many calories, which is why focusing on the markers of inflammation is the best dietary approach.

Diseases promoted by the metabolic syndrome

The metabolic syndrome is a chronic pro-inflammatory state, which is capable of pushing pro-inflammatory diseases into expression. The most notable conditions are cancer, diabetes, heart disease, heart attacks, stroke, hypertension, Alzheimer's disease, depression, osteoarthritis, tendinopathy, disc herniation, widespread pain, and back pain. Why is it that some people get cancer and others develop heart disease, or any of the other diseases listed above? We all have a genetic predisposition to develop various diseases, and if we live an inflammatory lifestyle, we nudge our genes to express their disease potential. This means that the metabolic syndrome is a pro-inflammatory state that pushes us into expressing the diseases that we are mostly genetically susceptible to develop. If someone has just musculoskeletal pain, people tend to just suffer through life. If depression develops too, this just adds to the misery of pain. If we are really unlucky, which is common, cancer may manifest. This is why we should all make sure our markers of inflammation are consistently normal.

The metabolic syndrome-fibrinogen-cancer connection

Fibrinogen is one of many substances that make up what is called connective tissue. There are two primary types of connective tissue substances, those being collagen and proteoglycans. Collagen is a fibrillar protein, which means that it is fibrous and gives a tissue its characteristic structure. In contrast to collagen, proteoglycans manifest as amorphous matrix, which is sometimes called ground substance. Collagen fibers and the ground substance made by proteoglycans, work together to give a tissue its characteristic form and shape. In other words, without connective tissue, our muscles and visceral organs would not have their characteristic structures that are easily identifiable in an anatomy lab.

Fibrinogen is one of several adhesive glycoproteins. In common language, this means that fibrinogen and other "sticky" connective tissue substances are also part of tissue stroma. The presence of fibrinogen helps cells to adhere and migrate to areas of tissue healing and unfortunately, also for pro-inflammatory/proliferative disease, such as tumor growth, atherosclerotic vascular disease (heart attack, stroke, and peripheral artery disease), Alzheimer's disease, and rheumatoid arthritis. Essentially any disease that is proliferative or expansive in nature is associated with elevated levels of fibrinogen.

Fibrinogen can be measured via a blood test and could have been included in the list of inflammation markers in *The DeFlame Diet* book. However, I chose not to add another layer of complexity in a general book about diet and inflammation. Fibrinogen is discussed in this book because it promotes breast cancer expression and the process by which fibrinogen promotes cancer is something we can visualize.

If you search the internet for the term "stroma," you will see that it is defined as the supportive tissue of an organ or *tumor*, which consists of connective tissue and blood vessels. You may also see terms used interchangeably with stroma, connective tissue and extracellular matrix. In short, solid tumors, as in breast cancer, require that stroma be present and proliferating; otherwise tumors cannot grow. Dr Dvorak first described this in 1986 and then again in 2015.[1,2]

It turns out that as early as 1998, scientists stated that elevated blood levels of fibrinogen, called hyperfibrinogenemia, should be considered a component of the metabolic syndrome.[3] Today, scientists are now describing elevated blood levels of fibrinogen to be a robustly correlated marker for the metabolic syndrome.[4,5] This is one of the reasons why people with the metabolic syndrome are more likely to develop the pro-inflammatory proliferative diseases listed above, including breast cancer.[6,7] Figure 1 below is a modification of Figure 1 from Chapter 2. It illustrates how fibrinogen is formed by the liver in response to the presence of pro-inflammatory cytokines, such as, interleukin-1 (IL-1) and interleukin-6 (IL-6)[8]

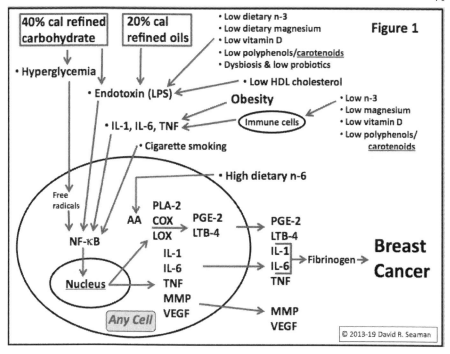

Figure 1

Not surprisingly, people with the metabolic syndrome tend to have elevated levels of these cytokines in circulation, and therefore, elevated fibrinogen.[4] But this appears to not be enough for breast cancer to proliferate aggressively. Breast tumor cells also produce fibrinogen, which reflects the importance of this "sticky" substance regarding tumor proliferation.[9] More recently, scientists identified that elevated preoperative blood levels of fibrinogen are associated with breast cancer progression and are independently associated with a poor prognosis in patients with operable breast cancer.[10] This means that circulating hyperfibrinogenemia is a strong promoter of breast cancer.

As illustrated above, it is important to remember that multiple contributing factors work together to create the pro-inflammatory state, which typically exists long before diseases develop, especially cancer. Consequently, people tend not to see the cause-effect relationship between diet and cancer expression. The reason is that the cause-effect relationship can actually take years to manifest, which is clearly the case of postmenopausal breast cancer expression.

The reason why understanding the relationship between a pro-inflammatory diet and fibrinogen is so important, is because as early as 1991, scientists hypothesized that the abundant fibrinogen present in the tumor connective tissue might contribute to the structural integrity of breast tumor tissues.[11] This was known 28 years ago, as of 2019, and I can assure you that moving forward, most people who develop breast cancer will unfortunately still be unaware of the metabolic syndrome-fibrinogen relationship to breast cancer. This is because the treatment of breast cancer, and other cancers, focuses on killing cancer cells and not on reducing the diet-induced pro-inflammatory state that promotes cancer and other chronic diseases.

Now that you know about the metabolic syndrome-fibrinogen relationship and the pro-cancerous nature of fibrinogen, you can be very proactive and do something. The goal should be to get all your inflammatory makers into the normal range, and if you want to get tested for fibrinogen, you can also do that for additional information to confirm the presence or absence of chronic inflammation.

References
1. Dvorak HF. Tumors: wounds that do not heal. Similarities between tumor stroma generation and wound healing. N Engl J Med. 1986;315:1650-59.
2. Dvorak HF. Tumors: wounds that do not heal—redux. Cancer Immunol Res. 2015;3:1-11.
3. Imperatore G, Riccardi G, Iovine C, et al. Plasma fibrinogen: a new factor of the metabolic syndrome. A population-based study. Diabetes Care. 1998;21:649-54.
4. Blaha M, Elasy TA. Clinical use of the metabolic syndrome: why the confusion. Clinical Diabetes. 2006;24:125-31.
5. Pinheiro Volp AC, Santos Silva FC, Bressan J. Hepatic inflammatory biomarkers and its link with obesity and chronic disease. Nutr Hosp. 2015;31:1947-56.
6. Porto LA, Lora KJ, Soares JC, Costa LQ. Metabolic syndrome is an independent risk factor for breast cancer. Arch Gynecol Obstet. 2011;284:1271-76.
7. Wani B, Aziz SA, Ganaie MA, Hussain MH. Metabolic syndrome and breast cancer risk. Indian J Med Paediatr Oncol. 2017;38:434-39.
8. Mei Y, Liu H, Sun X, et al. Plasma fibrinogen level may be a possible marker for the clinical response and prognosis of patients with breast cancer receiving neoadjuvant chemotherapy. Tumor Biol. 2017:1-7.
9. Simpson-Haidaris PJ, Rybarczyk B. Tumors and fibrinogen: the role of fibrinogen as an extracellular matrix protein. Ann NY Acad Sci. 2001;936:406-25.

10. Mei Y, Zhao S, Lu X, et al. Clinical and prognostic significance of preoperative plasma fibrinogen levels in patients with operable breast cancer. PLoS ONE. 2016;11(1):e0146233.
11. Costantini V, Zacharski LR, Memoli VA, et al. Fibrinogen deposition without thrombin generation in primary human breast cancer tissue. Cancer Res. 1991;51:349-53.

Chapter 10
Gut bacteria, breast bacteria, and breast cancer

The notion that "all diseases" arise from an unhealthy gut has been around for a long time. I first heard about this in 1982 when my career in healthcare began. To the untrained eyes and ears, the idea that the gut is the "root cause" of all diseases sounds appealing; however, it is a foolish notion. This statement suggests that the rest of the body remains healthy and normal until the gut crosses a critical "ill-health" threshold, which then spills into the rest of the body. In fact, the gut along with the rest of the body "flame up" together over time due to the consumption of excess refined sugar, flour, and oils.

Consider a young, healthy 20 year-old in the peak of health and vitality. Imagine that this person consumes a container of French fries, several pieces of bread, a cupcake (as illustrated on the cover of *The DeFlame Diet* book), and washes it down with soda or other sweetened beverage. Within 1-2 hours, there will be a blood sugar spike and a measurable rise in circulating bacterial endotoxin levels, which will lead to an immediate increase in circulating inflammatory chemicals.

The eating event described above will temporarily "flame up" the gut and the rest of the body. It should be understood that whenever we "flame" the gut, inflammation then occurs throughout the rest of the body.

To get a visual idea as to what happens to the gut and the rest of the body after engaging in a "drive-by self-shooting" event with dietary crack (refined sugar, flour, and oils), my suggestion is to watch my YouTube video entitled "The DeFlame Diet – Basics." The post-eating blood glucose and bacterial endotoxin surges are described in the video and more information about this process is described in *The Deflame Diet* book.

In short, it is impossible to create a healthy gut microbiota if excess refined sugar, flour, and oils are consumed. Important to understand is that we have varying degrees of tolerance to the consumption of these foods. Some can handle a lot without compromising gut and systemic (full body) health, while others are unable to tolerate much at all. You need to embrace whatever tolerance level you have and be respectful of it. In other words, do not make a habit of regularly breaching whatever your tolerance level happens to be.

A challenge to overcome is our general lack of appreciating the protracted nature of diet and chronic inflammation. It is very difficult for our minds to attach a cause-effect relationship to the dietary induction of inflammation because our brains witness us eating pro-inflammatory foods when we are young with no perceivable negative outcomes. Then, ten to twenty years later, we develop chronic pain, headaches, irritable bowel syndrome, or some other condition and we do not connect the dots to realize that our poor diets are causal. Furthermore, our emotional attachment to pro-inflammatory foods makes it difficult for the rational part of our brain to accept that foods we have loved for many, many years are the actual culprit.

What I just described in this paragraph is essentially the focus of my second book, *Weight Loss Secrets You Need To Know*. It is about understanding our biological, primordial, psychological and emotional relationship with food, and learning how to engage the rational part of our brain so that food no longer controls us.

A pro-inflammatory diet and our gut bacteria
Nothing more profoundly impacts the nature of our gut bacteria than our diet. For example, if we overeat refined sugar, flour, and oils, our gut bacterial species changes accordingly. Two distinct bacterial populations dominate our gut flora, those being a gram-negative group called Bacteriodetes and a gram-positive group called Firmicutes. Odds are you have never heard of either unless you read Chapter 15 in *The DeFlame Diet* book. These two species constitute at least 90% of all our gut bacteria.

While you probably did not know about Bacteriodetes and Firmicutes, it is quite likely that you have heard of lactobacillus acidophilus and bifidobacteria, and this is because each are popular supplements that are often advertised as being able to correct a gut bacterial imbalance. We do indeed need lactobacillus and bifidobacteria because they have many anti-inflammatory functions; however, when used as supplements, the outcomes can vary widely. For some people, they can be very helpful, but for many others, no perceivable benefit is derived. The reason for these different outcomes is that our diet exerts the primary control over the activity and balance of our gut bacteria. If you overeat refined sugar, flour, and oils and simultaneously eat very little vegetation, we depress the levels of both lactobacillus and bifidobacteria in our gut.[1,2] Supplementing with lactobacillus and bifidobacteria cannot restore the gut's bacterial balance to normal; the pro-inflammatory dietary drive that lowers these bacteria is too strong to be overcome by supplementation alone.

It is not uncommon for people to think that they need to have their specific bacterial population identified before making healthy changes; which typically involves a stool (poop) test. In fact, none of us need to do a stool test to get a basic understanding about whether our gut bacteria population is pro-inflammatory. Anyone eating the standard American diet that includes excess calories, most of which come from refined sugar, flour, and oils, will have a gut bacteria problem to varying degrees, which is mostly likely to be without significant symptoms, and can be rapidly corrected by DeFlaming the diet. When symptoms do occur from the gut, the most common reason is an overgrowth of bacteria in the small intestine, which is called small intestine bacterial overgrowth (SIBO), which in most cases can be dramatically improved, not surprisingly, by DeFlaming the diet. To help identify if you have a SIBO problem or a gluten problem, or both, read Chapters 14 and 15 in *The DeFlame Diet* book.

A pro-inflammatory diet and mammary gland/duct bacteria
It is important to understand that the human body contains more bacterial cells than human cells. Bacteria are all over us and within us

in certain locations, such as the mouth, the gut, urinary tract, vagina, and within the milk-producing apparatus of the breast. Essentially any part of the body that has contact with the environment to even a slight degree will have a bacterial population that can be disrupted by a pro-inflammatory diet. Consider that the cells of a milk-producing mammary gland and the duct system that conducts the milk to the nipple, are in contact with the outside world, which is how a baby is able to feed. This means that these areas of the breast are teeming with bacteria.

With the above information in mind, consider that a pro-inflammatory diet was associated with 10-fold reduction in mammary gland lactobacillus bacteria, compared to an anti-inflammatory diet.[1] This is quite relevant to breast cancer, as lactobacillus and other beneficial bacteria have the ability to break down carcinogens and decrease DNA damage.[3] Clearly, it is very important to eat an anti-inflammatory diet to deliver the proper bacteria to a nursing baby and to protect the breast against cancer expression.

Multiple studies have demonstrated a pro-inflammatory shift in the bacterial population within the breast of cancer sufferers.[1,4-6] In fact, there is a parallel shift within the bacteria of the gut and breast from one that is anti-inflammatory to pro-inflammatory, which is associated with breast cancer expression.[6] Unfortunately, microbiology is highly complex and trying to describe each bacteria is beyond my knowledge-base and the scope of this book. On a practical level, you need to know that a pro-inflammatory diet promotes a pro-inflammatory bacterial population within the gut and breast, which can help to promote breast cancer expression.

Here is additional motivation to DeFlame your diet to promote and maintain a healthy microbial environment in your body. Most people first experience true unconditional love and selflessness when they have children. Part of this experience should involve the delivery of the healthiest food possible to a newborn. With this in mind, consider the fact that the bacterial content of mother's milk is supposed to deliver lactobacillus, bifidobacteria, and other beneficial bacteria to the baby to promote the development of a normal bacterial population in the child.[7] Scientists recently stated that, "our results suggest that either the presence of lactobacilli and/or bifidobacteria or their DNA may constitute good markers of a healthy human milk microbiota."[8] Clearly, women need to be very careful to avoid an excess of pro-inflammatory calories if they want to provide their precious children with the most healthy breast milk possible, and simultaneously reduce the risk of developing breast cancer.

A pro-inflammatory microbiota and increased estrogen

As described earlier in this book, increased estrogen production promotes tumor expansion in most woman with breast cancer, and this is because breast cancers are estrogen positive or sensitive. It turns out that our gut bacterial population can function as a source of increased estrogen availability to breast cancer cells. Scientists have coined the term "estrobolome," which refers to the various bacteria that are capable of metabolizing estrogens.[9]

The term enterohepatic refers to the small intestine (entero) and the liver (hepatic). Enterohepatic circulation refers to a process by which the liver biochemically modifies drugs, bilirubin, hormones (such as estrogen), and other substances, which are released back into the small intestine, where they can be modified again by intestinal bacteria, and then these modified substances, such as estrogen, are either reabsorbed back into body circulation or they are eliminated in feces.

The enterohepatic circulation of estrogen is different among women, based on their diet. Strict vegetarians have increased fecal excretion of estrogens compared to non-vegetarians, leading to decreased estrogen concentrations in circulation, which means less estrogen can be delivered to breast cells. One study compared women who ate a pro-inflammatory, low fiber diet, with vegetarian women eating a high fiber diet. The vegetarian women had triple the amount of estrogen in feces and 15-20% lower blood levels of estrogen.[9]

With the above in mind, it is easy for some people to assume that they must be vegetarians in order to have healthy gut bacteria that do not deliver excess estrogen back into the body. It is a mistake to think this way, and equally foolish to think that eating animal fat is an independent driver of breast cancer. We know this because cancer in general and breast cancer specifically are rare in populations of people who eat their traditional natural foods and do not eat any refined sugar, flour, and oils. Examples include Eskimos who ate a high fat diet from sea and land animals, Masai people in Africa who eat meat, meat blood, and cows milk, and the Kitavans from New Guinea who eat mostly roots/tubers and fruit. These three very different populations are physically active, physically fit, and none traditionally consumed pro-inflammatory refined sugar, flour, and oils. This is why *The DeFlame Diet* can be very diverse, so long as these pro-inflammatory calories are avoided, and all the inflammatory markers are normalized.

References

1. Shively CA, Register TC, Appt SE, et al. Consumption of Mediterranean versus Western diet leads to distinct mammary gland microbiome populations. Cell Rep. 2018;25:47-56.
2. Sandhu KV, Sherwin E, Schellekens H, et al. Feeding the microbiota-gut-brain axis: diet, microbiome, and neuropsychiatry. Trans Res. 2017;179:223-44.
3. Malik SS, Saeed A, Baig M, et al. Anticarcinogenecity of microbiota and probiotics in breast cancer. Int J Food Prop. 2018;21:655-66.
4. Thompson KJ, Ingle JN, Tang X, et al. A comprehensive analysis of breast cancer microbiota and host gene expression. PLoS ONE. 2017;12(11):e0188873.
5. Urbaniak C, Gloor GB, Brackstone JM, et al. The microbiota of breast tissue and its association with breast cancer. Applied Environ Microbiol. 2016;82:5039-48.
6. Fernandez MF, Reina-Perez I, Astorga JM, et al. Breast cancer and its relationship with the microbiota. Int J Environ Public Health. 2018;15:1747.
7. Rodriguez JM. The origin of human milk bacteria: is there a bacterial entero-mammary pathway during late pregnancy and lactation. Adv Nutr. 2014;5:779-84.
8. Soto A, Martin V, Jimenez E, et al. Lactobacilli and Bifidobacteria in human breast milk: influence of antibiotherapy and other host and clinical factors. J Pediatr Gastroenterol Nutr. 2014;59:78-88.
9. Kwa M, Plottel CS, Blaser MJ, Adams S. The intestinal microbiome and estrogen receptor-positive female breast cancer. J Natl Cancer Inst. 2016;108:djw029.

Chapter 11
Epigenetics, methylation issues, folic acid, and breast cancer

The term epigenetics has gained a lot of traction and interest in recent years. Epigenetics refers to the modification of gene expression. Many articles have discussed epigenetics in the context of breast cancer:

> Romagnolo DF, et al. Epigenetics of breast cancer: modifying role of environmental and bioactive food compounds. Mol Nutr Food Res. 2016;60:1310-29.

> Pasculli B, et al. Epigenetics of breast cancer: biology and clinical implication in the era of precision medicine. Semin Cancer Biol. 2018;51:22-35.

The challenge we have to properly understand epigenetics involves the need to first understand genetics. This is typically where the so-called "wheels fall off" for many because genetics is a difficult field to grasp for most; it certainly was for me when I was in college. I found it much more confusing than physiology and biochemistry, so when I consider the topic of epigenetics, I look for a foundational concept to build my understanding.

It seems clear to me that the term epigenetics need not be used when describing how our genes express their genetic potential. Before the term epigenetics became popular, the terms genotype and phenotype were used to describe gene expression. Our genotype is hard wired; that is, we are disposed to express certain traits and diseases. In the case of disease expression, our genes typically place us at risk for developing disease. Just because we have certain gene risks for diseases does not mean that we will definitely express them. In most cases, we have to engage in pro-inflammatory behaviors for our genes to express disease. The term phenotype refers to the expression of disease. The best example of this that I have read involves the alleged relationship between red meat consumption and colon cancer expression.

Both authorities and bloggers typically tell us that eating red meat will increase our risk of developing colon cancer. In other words, in terms of genotype and phenotype, we are being told that eating red meat will cause our genes (genotype) to manifest colon cancer (the phenotype). If you search the internet for "epigenetics" you will see it is defined as, "the study of changes in organisms caused by modification of gene expression rather than alteration of the genetic code itself." So, using our colon cancer example, you can see that epigenetics really refers to the study of how red meat eating modifies gene expression of the genotype to promote colon cancer (a possible phenotype, that emerges due to eating red meat). In my opinion, no one needs to use the word epigenetics because in the context of disease expression, all it means on a practical level is that our lifestyle choices create a biochemical environment in our bodies that can induce our genotype to express an unwanted phenotype.

As stated above, we are told to not eat red meat if we want to avoid colon cancer. To better understand this relationship, scientists first identified if the subjects in the study had slow, intermediate, or rapid enzymes, called CYP1A2 and NAT2, which are involved in metabolizing carcinogens. They discovered that only the rapid metabolizers were more likely to get colon cancer, but in order for this to happen the subjects had to also be smokers and they had to eat well-done red meat. In other words, smoking and eating well-done red meat were the environmental stimuli required for the rapid enzymes (the genotype) to express the phenotype of colon cancer.[1] This also means that the broad recommendation to avoid red meat, because of the alleged cause-effect relationship between eating red meat and colon cancer, is a completely erroneous statement. In fact, in the study I just described, the rapid metabolizers were NOT at increased risk if they were non-smokers and they only ate red meat that was not well done. In other words, red meat promoted cancer only if it was eaten well done by smokers who were also rapid metabolizers. So, since I am not a smoker and I eat red meat that is medium rare or medium, I am not at risk of getting colon cancer from the red meat I eat.

Epigenetics and methylation

Methylation is a process that modifies gene expression. Methylation merely refers to adding a methyl group (CH_3) to your DNA to modify gene expression. The methylation of genes involved in cancer expression acts to turn off gene expression and inhibit the development of cancer. In contrast, when genes involved in cancer expression are not adequately methylated, they are not properly inhibited and so they are "released" to express cancer. What I just described is epigenetics. In the language of epigenetics, they would say that, "adequate methylation will epigenetically modify gene expression to prevent breast cancer." It turns out that folic acid metabolism is a key to proper methylation.

Folic acid and methylation

Folic acid is the term used to describe the type of vitamin B9 that is synthesized in the laboratory, which is referred to as synthetic folic acid. Folate or methyl-folate (CH_3–folate) are the abbreviated terms used to describe the vitamin B9 we find naturally in foods, which is most concentrated in green leafy vegetables. The actual name is 5-methyltetrahydrofolate, but we will use folate instead as it is easier to remember and is considered to be synonymous with 5-methyltetrahydrofolate. Note that "methyl" is part of the actual name for folate. The methyl group is what is transferred to DNA to prevent it from going rogue and allowing for the expression of cancer to occur. Before going any further, it should be understood that a lack of folate is just one of the many factors that adds to the pro-inflammatory state that drives cancer expression, so it needs to be thought of as part of the big "flame" that drives cancer and other diseases.

Folic acid and folate have different structures, with folate containing a methyl group (CH_3) that is lacking in the laboratory-synthesized folic acid. For orientation purposes, check out any multivitamin bottle or cereal box and you will see that folic acid, not folate, is typically used. When we consume folic acid, our body must convert it into folate before it becomes biologically active. The key enzyme involved in the activation of folic acid to folate is called methylene-tetrahydrofolate reductase or MTHFR for short, which converts *methylene*-tetrahydrofolate into the active **methyl**-tetrahydrofolate. There are variants or mutations of the MTHFR gene called polymorphisms; one is called C677T and the other is A1298C. Such polymorphisms may be a risk factor for breast cancer expression.[2,3]

According to the NIH, about 25% of Hispanics and 10-15% of Caucasians have C677T polymorphisms.[4] These numbers tend to scare people and are often used to scare people into doing expensive genetic workups. The "salespeople" physicians generally think that MTHFR polymorphisms are catastrophic and all people should be tested. In contrast, scientists are trying to work out the details to help provide a rational clinical approach to target the patients who should be tested. My take on this is straightforward.

If we lack an adequate amount of folate, we will not be able to convert a substance called homocysteine into another substance called methionine. So, the best way to identify if you have a folate problem is to do a blood test for homocysteine. If homocysteine is normal, we likely have nothing to worry about. If homocysteine is elevated, we may have a lot to potentially worry about. Elevated levels of homocysteine can promote multiple diseases, including atherosclerosis, chronic heart failure, bone fracture, Alzheimer's disease, dementia, stroke, carotid artery stenosis, deep-vein thrombosis, and increased total mortality and cardiovascular disease mortality.[5-9] Women with breast cancer are more likely to have high levels of homocysteine compared to those without the disease.[10,11]

A better homocysteine-methylation perspective to consider
Even with all of the abovementioned diseases in mind, elevated homocysteine does not mean that you have an MTHFR mutation. Multiple pro-inflammatory lifestyle issues can elevate homocysteine. A dietary deficiency of folate, high cholesterol, thyroid disease, diabetes, or unhealthy lifestyle factors (physical inactivity, smoking

and obesity), can all promote higher than normal levels of homocysteine.[4] If I had elevated homocysteine, I would DeFlame myself of the conditions listed above and this would obviously include a drastic increase in my consumption of folate-rich leafy greens, which we should all be doing anyway unless you are taking anti-coagulant medication, such as Coumadin/warfarin. I would also take a methyl-folate supplement. I would not initially test myself for a MTHFR polymorphism, because whether I had it or not, I would still do exactly what I mentioned in the last sentence. This is why it is not advisable to "freak out" about MTHFR mutations and epigenetics and make these more of an issue then they need to be.

To hopefully help put the homocysteine issue into even better perspective, consider the following study that was conducted on men and women ranging in age from 50-87. The authors wanted to see if taking a basic multivitamin/mineral supplement would impact homocysteine levels in the blood.[12] Most labs report normal homocysteine levels to be between 4-15 μmol/L, with an optimal level being below 10-12 μmol/L. A level between 15 and 30 μmol/L is considered mildly elevated, between 30 and 60 μmol/L is considered moderately elevated, and >60 μmol/L is considered severely elevated.[9] Elevated homocysteine levels are not uncommon; up to 5 to 7% of the general population has a mildly elevated homocysteine level. Individuals with the rare homocystinuria typically have blood levels of homocysteine that exceed 100 μmol/L.[9]

The average beginning homocysteine level in this study population was 9.5 μmol/L, so they were absolutely normal. The subjects took a multivitamin/mineral supplement that contained 2 mg of vitamin B6, 6 micrograms of vitamin B12, and 400 micrograms of "synthesized" folic acid. The study period was 56 days, after which the average homocysteine level dropped to 8.6 μmol/L.[12] This means that the synthesized folic acid used in this study had a beneficial effect, which is not uncommon if you look at other studies using folic acid. In fact, synthesized folic acid was used to fortify flours and in prenatal supplements because it reduced the incidence of neural tube defects.

I will explain at the end of this chapter how vitamins B6, B12, and folic acid relate to homocysteine levels.

With the above paragraphs in mind, you can hopefully see that living with fear about methylation, epigenetics, and homocysteine is not based on good evidence. Here is an additional perspective to consider. All of my grandparents and great grandparents lived to be in their late 80s to mid 90s. My one great aunt reached 100. None of them took B6, B12, and folic acid supplements, at least for any appreciable degree, which was the case for the vast majority of older people who lived most of their lives before vitamin supplements went mainstream and became popular. That generation of people was born in the late 1880s to about 1915, which is an important consideration. These people lived mostly on healthy natural foods, and they were alive long before deep-fried foods and sugar and flour became the predominant calorie sources in the American diet.

What is my point in the previous paragraph? My impression is that the homocysteine issue was pushed into being a bigger issue than it ever needed to be because Americans are sedentary and get most of their calories from desserts, snacks, and deep-fried food, which has caused multiple diseases and metabolic disturbances to have become more common to the point where they are accepted as normal…this is not normal. If these drastic lifestyle changes had not developed, my suspicion is that MTHFR polymorphisms and epigenetics, etc., would not have become an issue of heightened concern because most everyone used to be active and also ate adequate amounts of green vegetables that are rich in methyl-folate.

The folate-methylation-homocysteine cycle
There are 40 or more MTHFR polymorphisms. It seems that c677T and A1298C are the most relevant. The best evidence we have is that a polymorphism is only clinically relevant if it is promoting elevated levels of homocysteine – this could change as more is learned, but for now it appears that we should view polymorphisms not as polymorphisms specifically, but instead by assessing homocysteine levels. This perspective was clearly described in the journal

Circulation in 2005[8] and again in 2015.[9] Each paper is a free patient education piece, which can and should be read if you want more details about MTHFR mutations and homocysteine:

> Varga EA, Sturm AC, Misista CP, Moll S. Homocysteine and MTHFR mutations: relation to thrombosis and coronary artery disease. Circulation. 2005;111:e289-93.
> https://www.ahajournals.org/doi/pdf/10.1161/01.CIR.0 000165142.37711.E7
>
> Moll S, Varga EA. Homocysteine and MTHFR mutations. Circulation. 2015;132:e6-e9.
> https://www.ahajournals.org/doi/pdf/10.1161/CIRCUL ATIONAHA.114.013311

In the previous section, I mentioned that I would discuss vitamins B6, B12, and folate in the context of homocysteine levels. Figure 1 on the next page illustrates the folate-methylation-homocysteine cycle and how supplementation with folic acid and folate fit into the cycle.[13-17] Recall from above that CH_3 is called a methyl group. Whenever a CH_3 is transferred to another chemical, this transfer is called methylation.

Notice that CH_3–containing methionine is converted to S-adenosylmethionine (SAM), which transfers its CH_3 group so that DNA, RNA, and proteins can be methylated. This encapsulates the essence of what people are referring to when they talk about epigenetics, as described earlier in the above section entitled "Epigenetics and methylation."

As SAM gives up its CH_3 group, it is converted into SAH and then to homocysteine, which does not have CH_3 group. Notice that homocysteine is converted into methionine and cysteine by vitamin B6.

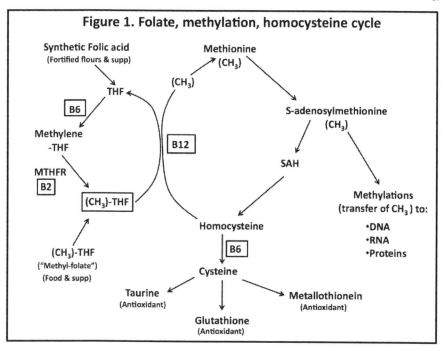

Figure 1. Folate, methylation, homocysteine cycle

Cysteine, which is considered to be an antioxidant amino acid, is used to make three important antioxidants, those being taurine, metallothionein, and glutathione (2GSH). Recall that glutathione was discussed in the free radical chapter. The conversion of homocysteine to three life-sustaining antioxidants, should alert us to the fact that homocysteine is a very important molecule; it should not be viewed as a solely pro-inflammatory substance. Not all homocysteine gets funneled into the cysteine pathway; the remainder must be converted back into methionine. If this does not happen, homocysteine will accumulate and cause the problems discussed earlier in this chapter.

To convert the excess homocysteine back to methionine, both vitamin B12 and methyl-folate, called methyl-tetrahydrofolate (CH₃-THF), are required. The terms methyl-folate and methyl-tetrahydrofolate are typically used interchangeably. Notice that we get methyl-folate from food, which adds CH3 to homocysteine to create methionine. In contrast, if we get synthetic folic acid, we need vitamin B6 to convert it to methylene-THF and then to methyl-THF. As described earlier, this conversion from methylene-THF to methyl-THF requires the MTHFR enzyme, which happens to require vitamin B2. If one has the MTHFR polymorphisms described earlier, they may not be able to convert methylene-THF to CH_3-THF, which means no CH_3 is available to add to homocysteine to make methionine.

In short, without CH_3-THF and vitamins B2, B6, and B12, this will cause homocysteine to accumulate and cause trouble. For perspective, despite the fact that way more than 5% of the general population have MTHFR polymorphisms, only approximately 5% of the general population has above normal homocysteine levels.[18] We don't know how many of these people have elevated homocysteine levels due to a MTHFR polymorphism or because of a pro-inflammatory lifestyle; however, it should be clear that only about 5% of the total population have elevated homocysteine levels and not everyone with elevated homocysteine has a MTHFR polymorphism as the cause. This should encourage people to develop a rational perspective about methylation issues and epigenetics.

Let's consider B12 for a moment. Most people with the metabolic syndrome or type 2 diabetes are treated with a drug called Metformin, which lowers B12 levels and can lead to elevated homocysteine levels.[19] Approximately 25% of the adult population has metabolic syndrome, which means a lot of people are taking a medication that promotes elevated levels of homocysteine. My suggestion is to get DeFlamed and eliminate the metabolic syndrome; however, if this cannot be achieved, vitamin B12 should be supplemented to the level needed to reduce homocysteine to normal.

It is also common for vegans to have high homocysteine levels. Vegans certainly get enough methyl-folate in their diet, but vitamin B12 is only found in animal products, the best sources being meat, dairy, and eggs.[20] For this reason, vegans should track their homocysteine levels and supplement with vitamin B12 as needed.

Potassium intake can influence homocysteine levels. Potassium was not discussed in this book; however, an entire chapter was devoted to potassium in *The DeFlame Diet* book, as it has multiple anti-inflammatory benefits and because very few Americans consume enough potassium. Researchers studied subjects with normal blood pressure who were salt sensitive, which means their blood pressure elevates when exposed to excess salt.[21] The subjects were loaded with salt, which caused their homocysteine levels to rise. This rise in homocysteine was prevented when the subjects were also given potassium. This does not mean that we should supplement with potassium. It is very important to get our potassium from food as described in *The DeFlame Diet*. Leafy green vegetables are the best source. See *The DeFlame Diet* book for more details.

Summary

The purpose of this chapter was to put epigenetics, methylation, and folic acid into perspective, because these topics will invariably come up if one looks outside of the traditional mainstream view of cancer expression. While this is an absolutely important clinical issue for some people, especially in the context of an MTHFR polymorphism, in no way is it the catastrophic problem it is made out to be in certain blogs, advertisements, websites, and YouTube videos. From the DeFlame perspective, your goal should be to normalize all the pro-inflammatory markers listed in Chapter 9 of *The DeFlame Diet* book, including homocysteine, if it happens to be elevated. Keep your head focused on normalizing the markers and do not let your mind get caught up in the nutritional drama that abounds.

References

1. Le Marchand L, Hankin JH, Wilkens LR, et al. Combined effects of well-done red meat, smoking, and rapid N-acetyltransferase 2 and CYP1A2 phenotypes in increasing colorectal cancer risk. Cancer Epidemiol Biomark Prev. 2001;10:1259-66.
2. Hosseini M, Houshmand M, Ebrahimi A. MTHFR polymorphisms and breast cancer risk. Arch Med Sci. 2011;7:134-37.
3. He L, Shen Y. MTHFR C677T polymorphism and breast, ovarian cancer risk: a meta-analysis of 19, 260 patients and 26,364 controls. OncoTargets Ther. 2017;10:227-38.
4. NIH. https://rarediseases.info.nih.gov/diseases/10953/mthfr-gene-mutation

5. McLean RR et al. Homocysteine as a predictive factor for hip fracture in older persons. New Eng J Med. 2004; 350:2042-49

6. Selhub J. The many facets of hyperhomocysteinemia: studies from the Framingham Cohorts. J Nutr. 2006; 136:1726S-30S.

7. den Heijer M et al. Hyperhomocysteinemia as a risk factor for deep-vein thrombosis. N Eng J Med 1996; 334:759-62

8. Varga EA, Sturm AC, Misista CP, Moll S. Homocysteine and MTHFR mutations: relation to thrombosis and coronary artery disease. Circulation. 2005;111:e289-93. https://www.ahajournals.org/doi/pdf/10.1161/01.CIR.0000165142.37711.E7

9. Moll S, Varga EA. Homocysteine and MTHFR mutations. Circulation. 2015;132:e6-e9. https://www.ahajournals.org/doi/pdf/10.1161/CIRCULATIONAHA.114.013311

10. Gatt A, Makris A, Cladd H, et al. Hyperhomocysteinemia in women with advanced breast cancer. Int J Lab Hematol. 2007;29:421-25.

11. Varela Almanza KM, Puebla-Perez AM Delgado-Saucedo JI, et al. Increased homocysteine plasma levels in breast cancer patients of a Mexican population. Exp Oncol. 2018;40:114-18.

12. McKay DL, Perrone G, Rsmussen H, et al. Vitamin/mineral supplementation improves plasma B-vitamin status and homocysteine concentration in healthy older adults consuming a folate-fortified diet. J Nutr. 2000;130:3090-96.

13. Scaglione F, Panzvolta G. Folate, folic acid and 5-methyltetrahydrofolate are not the same thing. Xenobiotica. 2014;44:480-88.

14. Crider Ks, Yang TP, Berry RJ, Bailey LB. Folate and DNA methylation: a review of molecular mechanisms and the evidence for folate's role. Adv Nutr. 2012;3:21-38.

15. Obeid R, Holzgreve W, Pietrzik K. Is 5-methyltetrahydrofolate an alternative to folic acid for the prevention of neural tube defects? J Perinat Med. 2013;41:469-83.

16. Troen AM, Lutgens E, Smith DE, et al. The atherogenic effect of excess methionine intake. Proc Nat Acad Sci. 2003;100:15089-94.

17. Ardawi MS, Rouzi AA, Qari MH, et al. Influence of age, sex, folate and vitamin B12 status on plasma homocysteine in Saudis. Saudi Med J. 2002;23:959-68.

18. Brustolin S, Giugliani R, Felix TM. Genetics of homocysteine metabolism and associated disorders. Braz J Med Biol Res. 2010;43:1-7.

19. Wile DJ, Toth C. Association of metformin, elevated homocysteine, and methylmalonic acid levels and clinically worsened diabetic peripheral neuropathy. Diabetes Care. 2010;33:156-61.

20. Elmadfa I, Singer I. Vitamin B-12 and homocysteine status among vegetarians: a global perspective. Am J Clin Nutr. 2009;89(suppl):1693S-98S.

21. Wan Z, Ren K, Wen W, et al. Potassium supplementation ameliorates increased plasma homocysteine induced by salt loading in normotensive salt-sensitive subjects. Clin Exp Hypertens. 2017;39:769-73.

Chapter 12
Iodine and breast cancer

Almost everyone focuses on the thyroid gland when they read or hear about iodine. In fact, breast tissue takes up iodine the way a dry sponge takes up water – not quite that dramatic; however, next to the thyroid gland, no other tissue appears to incorporate iodine in its structure as much as breast tissue during pregnancy and lactation. This led researchers to write the following article:

> Aceves C, Anguiano B, Delgado G. Is iodine a gatekeeper of the integrity of the mammary gland? J Mammary Gland Biol Neoplasia. 2005;10:189-96.

You might be wondering, why would the breast take up iodine the way it does? We can focus on two primary reasons. First, to provide iodine for a nursing infant. Second, iodine bonds to fatty acids (lipids) in cell membranes of the breast epithelial cells to form iodolipids called iodolactones, which protects them from becoming cancerous. These cell membrane fatty acids, such as arachidonic acid, are otherwise prone to become free radicalized, which means that iodine DeFlames the cell membranes of breast epithelial cells. With this in mind, consider that one of the risk factors for developing breast cancer is *never* being pregnant. I did not understand why that was the case, but thought it had something to do with lactation. Then I learned in the Aceves paper cited above, that during pregnancy and lactation, breast cells take up iodine from the blood supply more efficiently than the thyroid gland.

I then discovered that breast cancer is uncommon in Japanese women as a whole, whether they have children or not, because they eat more iodine than any other population. This made me realize that we can't really focus on pregnancy and lactation as the key reasons for less breast cancer in Japanese women. The issue appears to be more about adequate iodine intake in general and not because of the relationship between iodine uptake by the breast during pregnancy and lactation. We know this to be true because adequate iodine intake is not just an issue for breast cancer. Iodine also exerts its protective effect in the prostate gland and colon, to prevent prostate and colon cancer.[1,2] This means we all need to make sure we get enough iodine, but how much is enough?

Iodine intake in Japan

Whenever iodine intake is discussed, a comparison with Japan is always made because they consume a lot of iodine. So, how much iodine do Japanese women and men consume? If they eat a traditional diet consisting of seaweed and fish, iodine intake is thought to be about 1000-3000 micrograms (mcg) per day,[3] most of which comes from seaweed. The original estimates of Japanese iodine intake were up to 10,000 mcg or more, which was identified to be an overestimation after dietary intake was carefully accounted.[3]

Iodine intake in the United States

In the United States, the recommended intake for men and women 19 years and older is 150 mcg/day, which increases to 220 mcg for women during pregnancy and 290 mcg during lactation. Clearly, these values are well below the levels commonly consumed by the Japanese population; whether we go by the 1000 mcg, 3000 mcg, or the less likely, 10,000 mcg intake levels.

Seaweed provides the greatest amount of iodine on a caloric basis, which is not a staple in the American diet. Fish, shrimp, and other seafood provide the greatest amount of iodine in the American diet. For example, 3 ounces of cod, which is the size of a deck of cards, provides 99 mcg. Three ounces of shrimp provide 35 mcg. Standard portions of milk, yogurt, and cheese provide between 35-99 mcg. A medium baked potato with the skin delivers 60 mcg of iodine. You can see why the average American diet provides approximately 138-353 mcg/day.[4]

The upper limit in the US for individuals 19 years and older is 1,100 mcg/day. The US recommendations for most nutrients tend to err on the low side. For example, in Japan the upper limit is 3000 mcg/day;

however, it is not uncommon to exceed 3000 mcg without ill effect. So, in my mind, I default to laboratory testing for those who want to be absolutely sure about their iodine and thyroid status.

Testing iodine levels and thyroid function

About 90% of the iodine we consume is excreted in the urine, which means that it is difficult to reach an iodine toxicity level, unless one takes in extremely high amounts. However, there is another way one can develop iodine toxicity, which involves hypothyroidism that is caused by an autoimmune condition called Hashimoto's thyroiditis. People with Hashimoto's disease cannot tolerate as much iodine as those without the condition. Additionally, for certain people, eating or supplementing with too much iodine can push them into expressing Hashimoto's.

The best way to identify your iodine and thyroid status is to be tested. A typical blood test panel only looks at hormones related to thyroid function. To test for Hashimoto's thyroiditis, you would want to test for thyroid peroxidase (TPO) antibodies. A negative test means you do not have Hashimoto's thyroiditis.

ZRT Laboratory in Beaverton, Oregon has developed a simple blood spot test for thyroglobulin, thyroid stimulating hormones, thyroid hormones, and TPO antibodies. They have also developed a urine spot test for iodine, selenium, bromine, arsenic, mercury, and cadmium. Selenium is needed for the synthesis of thyroid hormones. Bromine, arsenic, mercury, and cadmium can compromise thyroid function and iodine/selenium status. ZRT also offers the iodine urine spot test by itself or along with selenium, bromine, arsenic, mercury, and cadmium.

The prevalence of Hashimoto's thyroiditis is .3-1.2%,[5] which means that no more than 1.2% of the US population has Hashimoto's. In other words, you have about a 1/100 chance of having the disease.

For patients with Hashimoto's thyroiditis, avoiding excess iodine is obviously very important. Additionally, many people derive benefit from taking 200 mcg of selenium, in the form of selenomethionine, which participates in thyroid hormone synthesis. This dose was effective in reducing TPO in patients with Hashimoto's thyroiditis after a 3-month period, compared with placebo.[6]

Individuals with Hashimoto's disease may derive benefit by eating a gluten-free diet.[7,8] This is because, in some cases, gluten withdrawal may single-handedly reverse Hashimoto's thyroiditis.[8]

Breast health studies with iodine supplementation
With the above cited intake levels in mind, studies have been done with iodine supplementation to help give us an insight about iodine tolerance and supplemental levels required to achieve a clinical benefit. In one study, 111 patients with cyclic mastalgia were treated with supplemental molecular iodine. Cyclic mastalgia is a painful condition of the breasts that is associated with the menstrual cycle. The breasts are tender and the pain is typically felt as a heavy dull ache, which may be associated with lumpiness.

The subjects in this study were supplemented with a placebo or 1500 mcg, 3000 mcg, or 6000 mcg of molecular iodine for three months.[9] It was a randomized, double-blind trial, which means that neither the subjects nor the physicians knew who was getting what. Here is the conclusion in the study:

> "Patients recorded statistically significant decreases in pain by month 3 in the 3000 and 6000 mcg/day treatment groups, but not the 1500 mcg/day or placebo group; more than 50% of the 6000 mcg/day treatment group recorded a clinically significant reduction in overall pain. All doses were associated with an acceptable safety profile. No dose-related increase in any adverse event was observed."

The outcome of this study provides us with important information. The supplemental dose, which is higher than the upper limit recommended by the United States and Japan, was associated with the best outcome and there were no associated side effects. This suggests that a large margin of tolerability exists for supplemental iodine.

Important to note is that I have seen cyclic mastalgia improve after women have DeFlamed without taking iodine supplements. This suggests that we should viewing DeFlaming as the most important thing one can do and to properly view supplements as "supplements" to *The DeFlame Diet*.

Iodine and estrogen

There are conflicting reports on the effects of iodine when applied to breast cancer cells in the laboratory. It is important to understand that cells in the lab are very different than cells in the body. Consider that it is possible to keep isolated cells alive in the lab for an indefinite period of time, so long as the nutritional environment is properly maintained. This was demonstrated by Dr. Alexis Carrel at the Rockefeller Institute of Medical Research in New York City beginning in 1912. This is in stark contrast to the cells that make up the human body...our cells are not isolated and maintained in a controlled environment. Cells in the human body are constantly being exposed to hormonal and nutritional changes during the aging process, which eventually leads to cell death and the death of the human body.

With the above in mind, in one study with breast cancer cells, iodine reduced estrogen receptor activity, which is preventive cancer expression.[10] In another study, iodine was shown to be stimulatory of the estrogen receptor, which promoted breast cell cancer expression.[11] While a stimulatory effect for iodine perhaps is the case for the laboratory model utilized in the latter study, it does not explain how the Japanese population, which consumes the most iodine on earth, has a very low breast cancer rate compared to the United States that consumes very much less iodine. I am far more inclined to view safe iodine levels based on the consumption pattern of the Japanese.

A potential complication for American women to consider

Just 3.5% of the Japanese population is obese compared to 35% of Americans. As you learned in Chapter 8, obesity is a risk factor for breast cancer and other chronic diseases. It is possible that the Japanese intake level of iodine may be protective only if you do not cross a certain body fat/weight threshold. Once that threshold is crossed, the effectiveness of iodine may diminish incrementally. I do not know if this is true or not; however, we must accept the fact that a 5'5" woman who weighs 120 pounds (BMI = 20) is very different biochemically (she is anti-inflammatory), compared to one who is the same height and weighs 190 pounds (BMI = 31.6) and is pro-inflammatory.

Final thoughts

This chapter about iodine should not be viewed as a treatment recommendation for Hashimoto's thyroiditis. The only reason for discussing this condition is because iodine supplementation is typically contraindicated in these patients. This means that if you have thyroiditis, you need to get it managed properly and need to be careful with an iodine supplement. A proper supplemental iodine dose can be correlated to TPO levels to make sure you are not pushing Hashimoto's into expression.

References

1. Aranda N, Sosa S, Delgado G, et al. Uptake and antitumoral effects of iodine and 6-iodolactone in differentiated and undifferentiated human prostate cancer cell lines. The Prostate. 2013;73;31-41.
2. Nava-Villalba M, Aceves C. 6-iodolactone, key mediator of antitumoral properties of iodine. Prostaglandins Other Lipid Mediat. 2014;112:27-33.
3. Zava TT, Zava DT. Assessment of Japanese iodine intake based on seaweed consumption in Japan: a literature-based analysis. Thyroid Research 2011;4:14.
4. NIH. https://ods.od.nih.gov/factsheets/iodine-healthprofessional/
5. Staii A, Mirocha S, Todorova-Koteva K, et al. Hashimoto's thyroiditis is more frequent than expected when diagnosed by cytology which uncovers a pre-clinical state. Thyroid Res. 2010;3:11.
6. Toulis KA, Anastasilakis AD, Tzellos TG, et al. Selenium supplementation in the treatment of Hashimoto's thyroiditis: a systematic review and meta-analysis. Thyroid. 2010;20:1163-73.
7. Jiskra J, Limanova Z, Vanickova Z, Kocna P. IgA and IgG antigliadin, IgA anti-tissue transglutaminase and antiendomysial antibodies in patients with

autoimmune thyroid diseases and their relationship to thyroidal replacement therapy. Physiol Res. 2003;52:79-88.

8. Satengna-Guidetti C, Volta U, Ciacci C, et al. Prevalence of thyroid disorders in untreated adult celiac disease patients and effect of gluten withdrawal: an Italian multicenter study. Am J Gastroenterol. 2001; 96(3):751-57.

9. Kessler JH. The effect of supraphysiologic levels of iodine on patients with cyclic mastalgia. Breast J. 2004;10:328-36.

10. Stoddard FR, Brooks AD, Eskin BA, Johannes GJ. Iodine alters gene expression in the MCF7 breast cancer cell line: evidence for an anti-estrogen effect of iodine. Int J Med Sci. 2008;5:189-96.

11. He S, Wang B, Lu X, et al. Iodine stimulates estrogen receptor signaling and its systemic level is increased in surgical patients due to topical absorption. Oncotarget. 2018;9:375-84

Chapter 13
Vitamin D and breast cancer

The issue of vitamin D deficiency has become extremely popular in the last 15-20 years. Research has identified that multiple diseases are promoted by a chronic deficiency of vitamin D. Table 1 below is from *The DeFlame Diet* book, which highlights many of the conditions related to a deficiency of vitamin D.

Table 1 - Potential consequences of vitamin D deficiency

Schizophrenia	Rickets
Depression	Osteomalacia (bone pain)
Metabolic syndrome	Widespread pain
Type 2 diabetes	Pseudofractures
Muscle weakness	Back pain
Muscle aches	Tuberculosis
Osteoporosis	Common cold
Osteoarthritis	Bacterial vaginosis
Influenza	Ulcerative colitis
Asthma	Rheumatoid arthritis
Cardiovascular disease	Parkinson's disease
Hypertension	Alzheimer's
Epilepsy	Breast cancer
Type 1 diabetes	Prostate cancer
Multiple sclerosis	Colon cancer
Crohn's disease	Pancreatic cancer

We now know for sure that there is an inverse association between vitamin D levels and breast cancer expression. This means that lower vitamin D blood levels are associated with an increased risk of breast cancer.[1] There are many mechanisms by which vitamin D exerts its anti-cancer effects. Recall from Chapter 2 and 3 that breast cancer arises in epithelial cells that line both the milk-producing lobules and the ducts that transmit milk to the nipple. If old epithelial cells are not targeted and eliminated as part of the normal cell death/replacement cycling process, which is referred to as apoptosis, normal cells can be transformed into malignant cells.

A lack of vitamin D also increases immune cell-mediated inflammation, which can promote cancer. There are many different types of immune cells. Figure 1 illustrates various T-lymphocytes. Th0 cells are T-helper precursor cells, which differentiate into T-helper 1 cells (Th1), T-helper 2 cells (Th2), T-helper 17 cells (Th17), and T-regulatory cells (Treg).

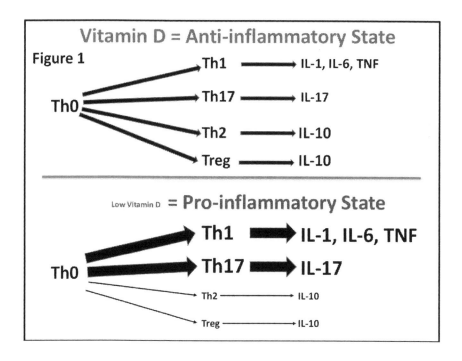

Th1 and Th17 cells promote inflammation by releasing pro-inflammatory cytokines, such as interleukin-1 (IL-1), interleukin-6 (IL-6), interleukin-17 (IL-17), and tumor necrosis factor (TNF). Th2 and Treg cells inhibit inflammation by releasing interleukin-10 (IL-10), the key anti-inflammatory cytokine. For a normal healthy anti-inflammatory state, we need a proper balance between the pro-inflammatory and anti-inflammatory cells and their respective cytokines. The balance is never shifted toward being too anti-inflammatory, which means the balance problem always shifts toward being pro-inflammatory. This means that we should not engage in behaviors that inhibit our anti-inflammatory T-cells to shift us into a pro-inflammatory state.

From a practical perspective, we can view any unhealthy lifestyle choice as a promoter of pro-inflammatory immune responses and an inhibitor of anti-inflammatory immune responses. This is obviously a very general statement and not so easy to visualize. Fortunately, vitamin D and immune cell function has been studied by scientists so we can create a visual image to never forget. Figure 1 illustrates what happens to immune cell expression when there is adequate and inadequate levels of vitamin D.[2-4]

Notice in Figure 1 that Th0 cells are the precursors to all the other T-cells. Th0 cells are referred to as naïve cells, which have the capacity to become both anti-inflammatory Th2 and Treg cells, or pro-inflammatory Th1 and Th17 cells. Notice that when there is adequate vitamin D, we get a balanced production of T-cells. However, when we are deficient in vitamin D, Th0 cells are converted into pro-inflammatory T-cells.

The pro-inflammatory and pro-cancer effects of the IL-1, IL-6, IL-17, and TNF have been described previously in this book, so I will not state them again. It is important to recall that the pro-inflammatory state of obesity and the metabolic syndrome mirrors the pro-inflammatory state created by a vitamin D deficiency. We also know that an inadequate intake of magnesium and omega-3 fatty acids supports vitamin D to promote the T-cell shift away from a pro-inflammatory state towards an anti-inflammatory state.[5,6] In other words, we suffer cumulative pro-inflammatory "hits" when we adopt an unhealthy lifestyle.

This is why the DeFlame approach to diet is about addressing and monitoring the inflammatory markers listed in the *The DeFlame Diet*. If we normalize all of the inflammatory markers, we have a much better chance of preventing and addressing chronic inflammatory conditions, such as breast cancer. In the context of this chapter, most experts agree that we should get our vitamin D tested, as measured by 25(OH)D in a blood test. The goal, as described in *The DeFlame Diet* book, should be to reach 70 ng/ml. Depending on sun exposure, it usually takes between 2000-10,000 IU of supplemental vitamin D3 to reach this level.

References

1. Atoum M, Alzoughool F. Vitamin D and breast cancer: latest evidence and future steps. 2017;11:11782234177.
2. Cantorna MT, Mahon BD. Mounting evidence for vitamin D as an environmental factor affecting autoimmune disease prevalence. Exp Biol Med. 2004; 229:1136-42.
3. Cantorna MT, Snyder L, Lin YD, Yang L. Vitamin D and 1,25(OH)2D regulation of T cells. Nutrients. 2015;7:3011-21.
4. Arnson Y, Amital H, Shoenfeld Y. Vitamin D and autoimmunity: a new aetiological and therapeutic considerations. Ann Rheum Dis. 2007;66:1137-42.
5. Chung HS, Park CS, Hong SH, et al. Effects of magnesium pretreatment on the levels of T helper cytokines and on the severity of reperfusion syndrome in patients undergoing living donor liver transplantation. Magnesium Res. 2013;26:46-55.
6. Hichami A, Grissa O, Mrizak I, et al. Role of T-cell polarization and inflammation and their modulation by n-3 fatty acids in gestational diabetes and macrosomia. J Nutr Metab. 2016; Article ID:3124960.

Chapter 14
Free radicals and breast cancer

Breast cancer, as well as other cancers and most other chronic diseases (heart disease, Alzheimer's, diabetes, osteoarthritis, etc.) are all states in which there is an excess of free radical activity. Free radicals are prominent players in the entire process of cancer development, from damage to the DNA molecule, the alteration of signaling pathways that promote cancer, and the regulation of progression of cancer.[1-9] This chapter will look at how free radicals are produced and how they are reduced. The lifestyle goal is to create a state that properly reduces and controls the expression of free radicals so they are no longer overproduced to participate in cancer expression. Figure 1 contains the basics about free radicals.

Figure 1. Antioxidant Defense

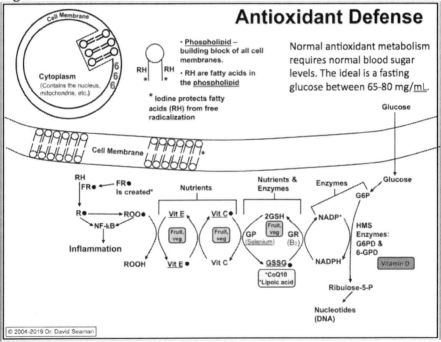

Most people have heard or read about free radicals. However, unless you study a good bit about body chemistry, it is difficult to conceptualize how free radicals are produced and then reduced by the body's antioxidant network. Years ago, I learned a way to visualize free radical activity in a simplified, yet biochemically accurate fashion to explain free radicals to those without science degrees. Table 1 below is the key for Figure 1 above.

Table 1. Key to Figure 1

Abbreviations	Descriptions
FR•	Free radical
RH	Fatty acid in phospholid, also called a lipid
R•	Fatty acid radical or lipid radical
ROO•	Lipid peroxyl radical
Vit E•	Vitamin E radical
Vit C•	Vitamin C radical
2GSH	Reduced glutathione (an antioxidant made by the body)
GSSG•	Oxidized or "free radicalized" glutathione
GP	Glutathione peroxidase (antioxidant enzyme that requires selenium)
GR	Glutathione reductase (antioxidant enzyme that requires riboflavin [vitamin B2])

The first thing you might notice is the cell in the top left with 666 in the cell membrane. The obvious Biblical reference notwithstanding, the 666 in this case refers to the overconsumption of omega-6 fatty acids that get inserted into cell membranes to create a pro-inflammatory state. We are supposed to consume a diet of less than a 4 to 1 ratio of omega-6 to omega-3 fatty acids in the diet, which was discussed in Chapter 3 in this book, and in several chapters in *The DeFlame Diet* book (Chapters 18, 25, 26). To the point of this chapter, an excess of omega-6 oil consumption promotes a state of free radical excess.[10] Ideally, the ratio of omega-6 to omega-3 should be 1:1; which would lead to a 6363 configuration in the cell membrane, which represents an anti-inflammatory state and non-cancerous state.

To the right of the cell is a blown-up image of a phospholipid. The circle represents what is called the phosphate head and the two vertical lines are fatty acids. It is important to understand that these fatty acids can be omega-6 or omega-3. The last thing we want is to load up our cell membrane phospholipids with omega-6 fatty acids at the expense of omega-3 fatty acids. Remember from Chapter 3 in this book that the average American eats a 10:1 to 25:1 ratio of omega-6 to omega-3, and this ratio should be less than 4:1 at worst; ideally as stated above, the ratio should be 1:1.

To the far right in Figure 1, it states that we need proper blood glucose levels in order to promote a proper free radical and antioxidant balance. Too much glucose in the blood supply leads to an excess production of free radicals, which cannot be controlled by dietary antioxidants or our body's antioxidant system.

Our antioxidant system involves both nutrients from our diet and our built-in antioxidant system that involves enzymes (which are a type of protein) that are a normal part of body function. In actual fact, nutrients and enzymes work together to keep free radical production at a healthy level.

The problem that most people have when it comes to understanding antioxidants and free radicals, is that they do not understand that supplementation cannot fix the antioxidant enzyme system. In other words, overeating refined sugar, flour, and omega-6 oils creates a perpetual free radical state; in part by nutrient deficiency, but also by altering the normal function of our antioxidant enzyme system that favors an excess of free radicals. This means that the most important antioxidant activity we can engage in is the elimination of excess calories from refined sugar, flour, and oils. Consider also that overeating these calories leads to obesity and type 2 diabetes, both of which are inflammatory states that are associated with an excess production of free radicals,[8,9,11] which goes on 24 hours per day in an unrelenting fashion. It is important to understand that overeating refined sugar, flour, and omega-6 oils creates a state wherein free radicals are perpetually overproduced, which cannot be corrected by supplements, which means we must DeFlame the diet.

Notice in Figure 1 that [Fruit,Veg] is listed three times. The reason is that the polyphenols and carotenoids in vegetation represent our natural source of antioxidants. We also get polyphenols from various spices that are also used as supplements, the most notable being ginger and turmeric.

It is important to understand that free radicals are created constantly in the body by virtue of our dependency on oxygen to survive. Imagine that you bite an apple and let it sit on your counter. Within a short period of time, the flesh exposed to the air by the bite will begin to turn brown. This is called oxidation and in the human body, such oxidation refers to free radical production. If you were to take two bites on opposite sides of the apple and squeeze lemon juice on one side, you will notice that it does not oxidize as quickly. This is because lemons contain antioxidants that prevent oxidation. Our goal with diet and supplements is to keep free radical production at a normal level.

On the far left in Figure 1, you can see that a free radical is created and attacks a fatty acid in the cell membrane to create a lipid radical, which can be converted into a lipid peroxyl radical. Both of these free radicals can stimulate NF-kB to stimulate ongoing inflammation. To the immediate right of these free radicals you can see vitamins E and C, which are specific nutrients that can reduce lipid and lipid peroxyl radicals. This is the extent to which most people think about free radicals and antioxidants.

Notice what happens to Vitamin E after it reduces the lipid peroxyl radical...Vitamin E now becomes a free radical. Vitamin C then comes along and reduces the vitamin E radical. But now vitamin C becomes a free radical, and 2GSH must come to the rescue, which involves both nutrients and enzymes.

As stated in Table 1, 2GSH is called reduced glutathione, which is a special antioxidant that our bodies make from three amino acids called cysteine, glycine, and glutamic acid. Enzymes in our body are responsible for building glutathione from the three amino acids. The enzyme glutathione peroxidase, which requires selenium, utilizes 2GSH to reduce the vitamin C radical back to its normal antioxidant vitamin C. But now 2GSH is radicalized into GSSG• and must be reduced back into 2GSH. This requires the enzyme glutathione reductase (GR), which requires riboflavin (vitamin B2) and NADPH. Supplemental lipoic acid and CoQ10 can assist in the process of reducing GSSG• back into 2GSH.

We need proper blood glucose levels to produce NADPH from NADP, which is why maintaining a proper blood glucose level is the most important thing we can do to keep free radical production in the normal range. There are two enzymes (GSPD and 6-GPD) involved in the production of NADPH, which require vitamin D to function properly. NADPH is not something we get from diet or supplements; we must produce adequate levels of NADPH in our bodies, as it is the key antioxidant that supports our body's entire antioxidant system.

Notice also in Figure 1 that iodine protects fatty acids from being radicalized. This topic was discussed in Chapter 12.

Alcohol and breast cancer
It turns out that an excess of alcohol consumption leads to an increased production of free radicals (2), which we clearly do not want. My perception is that 1-2 drinks per day, or a few times per week, referred to as moderate alcohol consumption, should not be viewed as a risk factor for breast cancer expression or any other disease, as long as one is eating an anti-inflammatory diet. However, you would not get this impression if you spent some time on the internet.

If you were to search the internet for "alcohol and breast cancer," multiple scientific studies will appear that link alcohol consumption to breast cancer expression. You will see that moderate drinking is claimed to be associated with a 30-50% increase in risk of developing breast cancer. Clearly, these numbers can look scary in terms of percentages; however, this can be misleading because of the statistics that are utilized. I fabricated the following numbers so you understand the difference between relative risk and absolute risk. Studies that report statistical risk almost exclusively utilize relative risk, which is a statistical method that is NEVER considered by the average person.

Imagine that 10,000 moderate drinkers were compared to 10,000 non-drinkers to identify cancer risk associated with moderate alcohol consumption. In the drinker group, 200 developed breast cancer, while in the non-drinker group, only 100 developed breast cancer. If you consider this from the perspective of absolute risk, there is only a 1% difference in risk. This is because 200 people out of 10,000 drinkers represents 2%, which means that 98% of moderate drinkers did NOT develop breast cancer. In the case of 100 cancer cases out of 10,000 people, this means that 1% of non-drinkers developed breast cancer, while 99% did not. Clearly, using the common math that non-scientists use, this means there is only a 1% difference. What do you think happens if you do the math using relative risk?

When percentages are reported based on relative risk, the number of subjects (10,000 in our example) is ignored. The statistical focus is directed solely at the 200 cases of breast cancer in the moderate drinker category and 100 cancers in the non-drinkers. The number 100 is 50% less than 200, which allows for the conclusion, based on relative risk, that moderate drinking leads to a 50% greater risk of developing breast cancer. However, if we use common math, we know that the difference is actually only 1%. I am personally not worried about a 1% difference in risk for developing any disease.

With the above in mind, if you look at risk based on percentages, unless otherwise stated, the scientists are using relative risk. Sometimes scientists do, in fact, state that they are comparing disease expression based on relative risk, which they did indicate in the body of this paper that also stated the following in the introduction:[12]

> "Extensive epidemiologic data have linked alcohol consumption to risk of breast cancer. The overall

> estimated association is an approximate 30-50% increase in breast cancer risk from 15-30 grams/day of alcohol consumption (about 1-2 drinks/day)."

First, it is important to recognize that the authors say extensive data connects alcohol to breast cancer. If we view this from the perspective of absolute risk, I would disagree and I would not be concerned about moderate alcohol consumption. Using our example of 10,000 subjects, a 30% percent increased risk translates into 140 breast cancer cases out of 10,000 moderate drinkers and 200 cases out of 10,000 non-drinkers. This is less than a 1% difference when common math, that we all understand, is used, which again is called absolute risk in the odd land of scientific statistics.

Second, what scientists rarely if ever do is consider the risk potential of alcohol in the context of the average American's diet, which consists of 60% of calories from refined sugar, flour, and omega-6 oils. My perception is that if normal body weight is maintained by eating an anti-inflammatory diet, AND less than 10% of calories per day came from refined sugar, flour, and omega-6 oils, there would be virtually no risk of breast cancer from a couple of drinks per day. This would especially be the case if red wine and/or stout beer were consumed, each of which contains anti-inflammatory polyphenols that are anti-inflammatory. The reason why I am confident about this is because of a revealing study on subjects with the metabolic syndrome who were allowed to consume alcohol as part of their diet.

Scientists in Spain had patients with the metabolic syndrome eat a diet that was free of refined sugar, flour, and oils, and also free of grains, legumes, fruit, and potatoes. The study subjects ate vegetables, fish, cheese, meat, olive oil, and moderate red wine. They did this for three months, at which time all subjects who followed the program were free of the pro-inflammatory metabolic syndrome.[13] In other words, moderate alcohol consumption did not have a pro-inflammatory effect when consumed with a DeFlaming diet.

I am not suggesting that you should drink alcohol; rather I am suggesting that moderate alcohol consumption is not going to push the average person into a breast cancer state. Heavy drinking could do it and moderate drinking along with a pro-inflammatory diet could do it as well. However, moderate alcohol consumption in addition to an anti-inflammatory diet is not likely to have any breast cancer-promoting effect.

Summary

This chapter painted a picture of free radicals to help you better understand that free radicals cannot be counteracted merely by taking vitamins E, C and selenium. This is because overeating refined sugar, flour, and oils produces excess free radicals, and this occurs whether you are young and healthy or old and not so healthy. Additionally, this same pattern of eating, over time, leads to the development of obesity and diabetes, both of which represent chronic inflammatory states that are characterized by an excess of free radical production 24 hours per day, whether one is eating or sleeping. With obesity and/or diabetes, the consumption of refined sugar, flour, and oils only serves to acutely increase free radical production to an even higher level. Eventually, the outcome will be a more devastating chronic disease, such as breast cancer.

So our antioxidant plan, which applies to everyone in my opinion, should be to drastically reduce the consumption of refined sugar, flour, and omega-6 oils; increase our consumption of vegetation; and normalize our body weight and all the inflammatory markers outlined in Chapter 9 of *The DeFlame Diet* book. Consider adding an iodine supplement to the daily routine. Supplementation with CoQ10, vitamin D and omega-3 fish oils is also a good idea. I personally take these four supplements every day in addition to the others I listed in Chapter 30 in *The DeFlame Diet* book.

References
1. Noda N, Wakasugi H. Cancer and oxidative stress. J Japan Med Assoc . 2001;44:535-39.
2. Saha SK, Lee SB, Won J, et al. Correlation between oxidative stress, nutrition, and cancer initiation. Int J Mol Sci. 2017;18:1544.

3. Brown NS, Bicknell R. Hypoxia and oxidative stress in breast cancer. Oxidative stress: its effects on the growth, metastatic potential and response to therapy of breast cancer. Breast Cancer Res. 2001;3:323-27.

4. Jezierska-Drutel A, Rosenzweig SA, Neumann CA. Role of oxidative stress and the microenvironment in breast cancer development and progression. Adv Cancer Res. 2013;119:107-25.

5. Junior AL, Paz MF, da Silva LI, et al. Serum oxidative stress markers and genotoxic profile induced by chemotherapy in patients with breast cancer: a pilot study. Oxidative Med Cell Longevity. 2015; Article ID 212964.

6. Hecht F, Pessoa CF, Gentile LB, et al. The role of oxidative stress on breast cancer development and therapy. Tumor Biol. 2016;37(4):4281-91

7. Mencalha A, Victorino VJ, Cecchini R, Panis C. Mapping oxidative changes in breast cancer: understanding the basic to reach the clinic. Anticancer Res. 2014;34:1127-40.

8. Hakkak R, Korourian S, Melnyk S. Obesity, oxidative stress and breast cancer risk. J Cancer Sci Ther. 2013;5(12):1000e129.

9. Kruk J. Overweight, obesity, oxidative stress and the risk of breast cancer. Asian Pac J Cancer Prev. 2014;15:9579-86.

10. Berry EM. Are diets high in omega-6 polyunsaturated fatty acids unhealthy? Eur Heart J Suppl. 2001;3(Supplement d):D37-D41.

11. Ullah A, Khan A, Khan I. Diabetes mellitus and oxidative stress—a concise review. Saudi Pharmaceutical J. 2016;24:547-553.

12. McDonald JA, Goyal A, Terry MB. Alcohol intake and breast cancer risk: weighing the overall evidence. Curr Breast Cancer Rep. 2013 Sep;5(3).

13. Perez-Guisado J, Munoz-Serrano A. A pilot study of the Spanish ketogenic Mediterranean diet: An effective therapy for the metabolic syndrome. J Med Food. 2011;14:681-87.

Chapter 15
Omega-6 fatty acids and breast cancer

Omega-6 fatty acids have been mentioned or discussed in Chapters 1, 2, 3, 5, 6, and 14 of this book. I chose to include this short chapter for the purpose of emphasizing how important it is to avoid consuming an excess amount of omega-6 fatty acids for the purpose of preventing breast cancer expression.

A key point to understand about omega-6 (n-6) fatty acids is that they are one of many pro-inflammatory risk factors that we should all be concerned about, but in a rational way. I say this because in various books and blogs, n-6s are dramatized to such a degree that it makes people terrified to eat a donut or French fry ever again, for fear of that meal causing cancer or heart disease in that moment. Here is a better perspective...

We have known for several decades that overeating omega-6 fatty acids is promotional for breast cancer and other chronic diseases. The key word in the previous sentence is "overeating." We are supposed to get close to an equal balance of omega-6 and omega-3 fatty acids in our diet, which means that we absolutely need omega-6 fatty acids...just not an excessive amount.

We can easily avoid an excess of omega-6 fatty acids by avoiding packaged snacks and deep-fried foods, and by never using omega-6 oils when cooking at home, including corn, safflower, sunflower, peanut, soybean, and grapeseed oils. In addition to avoiding the n-6 foods and oils, taking about 1000-3000 mgs of omega-3s (EPA/DHA) from a fish oil supplement is a typical recommendation, which I agree with. For more details about fatty acids in food and supplements, there are fifty pages of information in *The DeFlame Diet* book. In the meantime, here is some motivation to help you avoid an excess of omega-6 fatty acids in the context of breast cancer.

When scientists add omega-6 fatty acids to breast cancer cells in the laboratory, the cells become aggressive and invasive.[1-3] In contrast, when breast cancer cells are cultured with omega-3 fatty acids, their growth is inhibited.[3] In a recent animal study, breast cancer cells were implanted in mice. In the mice that were fed the higher omega-3 diet, there was a significant delay in tumor growth initiation and a prolonged survival time compared to those on the lower omega-3 diet.[4] A similar finding has been identified in human females. A pathological shift in breast cells that predispose one to develop cancer is called cytologic atypia.[5] Not surprisingly, women who consumed more omega-3 fatty acids had less atypical changes in breast cells, reflecting a tumor suppressive effect.

It should be noted that supplemental omega-3 fatty acids from fish oil do indeed become incorporated into breast cells.[6] While this is quite desirable, it is very important to understand that, as a single approach, fish oil supplementation alone will not lead to a robustly healthy state of body chemistry, which is needed to prevent breast cancer and other chronic diseases. This is why addressing all of the pro-inflammatory factors listed in this book and normalizing all of the inflammatory markers outlined in *The DeFlame Diet* is the best approach to take for all of your family members.

References

1. Villegas-Comonfort S, Castillo-Sanchez R, Serna-Marquez N, et al. Arachidonic acid promotes migration and invasion through a PI3K/Akt-dependent pathway in MDA-MB-231 breast cancer cells. Prostaglandins Leukot Essent Fatty Acids. 2014;90:169-77.
2. Serna-Marquez N, Diaz-Aragon R, Reyes-Uribe E, et al. Linoleic acid induces migration and invasion through FFAR4- and PI3K-/Akt-dependent pathway in MDA-MB-231 breast cancer cells. Med Oncol. 2017;34:111.
3. MacLennan M, Ma Dw. Role of dietary fatty acids in mammary gland development and breast cancer. Breast Cancer Res. 2010;12:211.
4. Khadge S, Thiele GM, Sharp JG, et al. Long-chain omega-3 polyunsaturated fatty acids decrease mammary tumor growth, multiorgan metastasis and enhance survival. Clin Exper Metasasis. 2018;35:797-818.
5. Hidaka BH, Li S, Harvey KE, et al. Omega-3 and omega-6 fatty acids in blood and breast tissue of high-risk women and association with atypical cytomorphology. Cancer Prev Res. 2015;8:359-64.

6. Bagga D, Capone S, Wang HJ, et al. Dietary modulation of omega-3/omega-6 polyunsaturated fatty acid ratios in patients with breast cancer. J Natl Cancer Inst. 1997;89:1123-31.

Chapter 16
Fasting and breast cancer

Fasting has become a very popular topic in recent years, during the same time that the ketogenic diet has become popular again. I say "popular again" because *The Atkins Diet*, which has been around for years, is a ketogenic diet.

Fasting should be the least confusing of all dietary issues for us to wrap our minds around, since it involves eating no food at all. No one needs to be confused about what NOT to eat…we should simply eat nothing and drink water during the fasting period.

The easiest fasting approach to engage in is called time-restricted feeding. A study was published in 2016 that looked at time-restricted feeding in the context of breast cancer recurrence. Women who fasted for 13 hours or more had a reduced risk of breast cancer recurrence compared to those who fasted less than 13 hrs.[1] Not surprisingly, the beneficial effect of time-restricted feeding is better blood glucose regulation, which means lower fasting glucose and lower hemoglobin A1c, which is a marker of long term (3 months) glucose control. In the context of breast and other cancers, the last thing one wants is hyperglycemia, which can readily feed cancer cells as described earlier in this book.

My personal feeling is that we should all do a nightly fast of at least 13 hours, with the ultimate goal being 16 hours or longer.[2] This means that our eating window should be 8 hours. If your last eating event is at 8 PM, your next eating event should be at 12 noon or later…it is that simple. I do not always achieve 16 hrs, but I always go for at least 13 hrs.

If you restrict eating for 13 hours, then your feeding period or eating window is 11 hours. If you restrict eating for 16 hours, then your eating window is 8 hours. During the feeding time period, the goal should obviously be to consume the foods listed in *The DeFlame Diet* or the The DeFlame Ketogenic Diet, and avoid pro-inflammatory calories…it is that simple.

Pro-inflammatory vs. DeFlame Diet vs. DeFlame Ketogenic Diet

Pro-inflammatory calories	DeFlame Diet	DeFlame Ketogenic Diet
Refined sugar	Grass-fed meat and wild game	Grass-fed meat and wild game
Refined grains	Meats	Meats
Grain flour products	Wild caught fish	Wild caught fish
Trans fats	Shellfish	Shellfish
Omega-6 seed oils (corn, safflower, sunflower, peanut, etc.)	Chicken	Chicken
	Omega-3 eggs	Omega-3 eggs
	Cheese	Cheese
	Vegetables	Vegetables
	Salads (leafy vegetables)	Salads (leafy vegetables)
	Fruit	* No fruit
	Roots/tubers (potato, yams, sweet potato)	* No roots/tubers
	Nuts (raw or dry roasted)	Nuts (raw or dry roasted)
	Omega-3 seeds: hemp, chia, flax seeds	Omega-3 seeds: hemp, chia, flax seeds
	Dark chocolate	* Sugar free dark chocolate
	Spices of all kinds	Spices of all kinds
	Olive oil, coconut oil, butter, cream, avocado, bacon	Olive oil, coconut oil, butter, cream, avocado, bacon
	Red wine and dark beer	Red wine
	Coffee and tea (green tea is best option)	Coffee and tea (green tea is best option)
		* No legumes and whole grains

As stated previously in Chapter 5 of this book, a state of ketosis is most desirable for the purpose of "starving" cancer cells of the glucose they need to grow. This means that eating a ketogenic diet in a time-restricted feeding window is the most biologically advantageous approach to anti-inflammatory eating.

As described earlier in Chapter 7, a 66-year old woman was diagnosed with recurrent breast cancer and was scheduled for surgery in three weeks.[3] The pre-surgical biopsy was both estrogen receptor positive and also positive for HER2. Immediately upon receiving the diagnosis, the woman began a strict ketogenic diet and also supplemented with 10,000 IU of vitamin D3. After the tumor was removed, it was tested again and found to be no longer positive for HER2, and this improvement occurred in just three weeks. While this excellent outcome is limited to a single case history, it should not dissuade us all from pursuing and maintaining a DeFlamed state of body chemistry.

References
1. Marinac CR, Neslon SH, Breen CI, et al. Prolonged nightly fasting and breast cancer prognosis. JAMA Oncol. 2016;2:1049-55.
2. Moro T, Tinsley G, Bianco A, et al. Effects of eight weeks of time-restricted feeding (16/8) on basal metabolism, maximal strength, body composition, inflammation, and cardiovascular risk factors in resistance-trained males. J Translation Med. 2016;14:290.
3. Branca JJ, Pacini S, Ruggiero M. Effects of pre-surgical vitamin D supplementation and ketogenic diet in a patient with recurrent breast cancer. Anticancer Res. 2015;35:5525-32.

Chapter 17
Breast cancer chemistry is similar to autism chemistry

Why autism is in a book about breast cancer

Physicians and the general public have been conditioned to view diseases as being individual distinct entities that should be targeted with medications. As I outlined in *The DeFlame Diet* book, this mental conditioning has created a false reality about how to look at health and disease. While different diseases certainly have different symptoms, the underlying cause is nearly identical, that being a chronic pro-inflammatory state, which happens to be the case for breast cancer, autism, and essentially every other disease that people have or are worried about getting. Figure 1 below, which I first presented in Chapter 10 in *The DeFlame Diet* book, illustrates what you just read in the last sentence. The center circles reflect the pro-inflammatory state, which serve as the promoters of all the diseases listed in the outer circle.

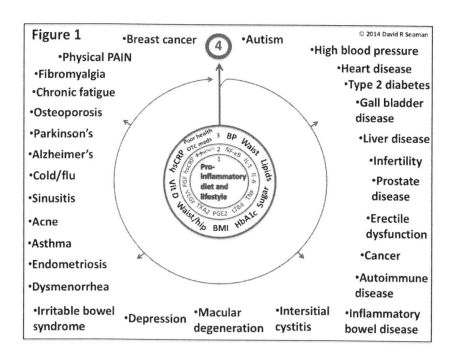

Since breast cancer chemistry is essentially identical to autism chemistry, I decided to include this chapter for the purpose of motivating parents to become as healthy as possible before conceiving a child. By doing this, not only does the woman reduce her risk of developing breast cancer and other chronic diseases, she also profoundly reduces her risk of having an autistic child.

Autism statistics

The CDC says that 1 in 68 children currently have autism spectrum disorder, while in the 1960s and 1970s, according to the National Institutes of Health; the prevalence was estimated to range from 1/2500 to 1/5000. It is certainly possible that the prevalence could have been greater, based on diagnostic criteria and reporting procedures utilized in the 60s and 70s. Either way, there is no disagreement within the scientific community that autism is far more common now compared to those early years. I can say that as a child growing up in the 60s and 70s, we had no idea what autism was. Only the extremely rare child had Down syndrome and a few kids had dyslexia.

One of the emerging risk factors for autism is aging, which scientists refer to it as inflammaging.[1-4] Compared to now, in the mid 20th century and earlier, parents typically had children in their early 20s. Now people commonly wait until they are in their mid to late 30s or older, which is an issue of inflammatory concern. All you need to do is look at the average 22 year-old man or woman and compare them to 35 year-olds. The 22 year-olds look like kids compared to the 35 year-olds. The odds that people are going to start having children when they are in their early 20s anytime soon is quite unlikely. This is primarily due to the economic challenges that young people now face, and the desire for women to put off having children until after they pursue a career. This is why anyone planning on having kids needs to adopt a DeFlaming lifestyle as early as possible and maintain a DeFlamed state throughout their lives to protect themselves and future offspring against inflammatory diseases listed in Figure 1.

Autism as an autoimmune-type of condition

The debate about whether or not vaccines can cause autism has served to muddy the water, such that the average person has no idea what autism actually is. In fact, multiple studies have characterized the chemistry of autism to be consistent with that of other autoimmune diseases.[5-11] Not surprisingly, there is an increased risk of autism expression in the offspring of parents with autoimmune diseases.[11]

Autoimmune diseases are a category of conditions in which the immune system attacks and damages our own body tissues. Perhaps the most well-known autoimmune disease is rheumatoid arthritis. Additional classical autoimmune diseases include psoriasis, systemic lupus erythematosus, ankylosing spondylitis, scleroderma, Sjogren's Syndrome, and temporal arteritis.

The unifying feature of all autoimmune diseases involves an immune system shift from one that is non-inflammatory and healing to one that is pro-inflammatory and misperceives body tissue as a foreign invader that needs to be attacked. The obesity chapter in this book illustrated the pro-inflammatory shift in immune function as one goes from a lean to an obese state. While the obesity immune profile reflects an autoimmune state, this does not mean that all obese people will develop an autoimmune disease. Multiple factors are required for an autoimmune disease to express itself.

In 2000, an article outlined the factors associated with the expression of rheumatoid arthritis, which included genes, infections, stress system activation, and excess production of female hormones.[12] Save for female hormone excess, genetics, infections, and stress are all promoters of autism. It turns out that autism is promoted by nearly identical pro-inflammatory changes in the mother and her offspring, as will be described in the remainder of this chapter.

Maternal inflammation and autism

Chapter 7 outlined how obesity can promote breast cancer and Chapter 8 outlined how the metabolic syndrome and diabetes can promote breast cancer. Not surprisingly, studies have shown that maternal obesity and diabetes promote autism in offspring.[13,14] Scientists have identified that pre-pregnancy obesity places a child at risk for many developmental disorders, including autism spectrum disorder, attention deficit-hyperactivity disorder, developmental delay, and emotional/behavioral problems.[13-15] Why would this be the case, you may ask? You have to remember from Chapter 7 that the pro-inflammatory state of obesity is similar to autoimmune chemistry. This means that the little developing brain of the fetus is bathed in autoimmune-like chemistry for 9 months; so, it should not be a surprise that this would place the child at risk for developing a mental disorder such as autism, which is a manifestation of autoimmune chemistry.

Figure 1 below is the obesity image from Chapter 7. Notice the inflammatory chemicals that are pumped out into circulation by the pro-inflammatory immune cells that associate with obese fat cells, all of which can "flame up" the brain of the developing fetus. Take special notice of IL-17, which is produced by Th17 cells.

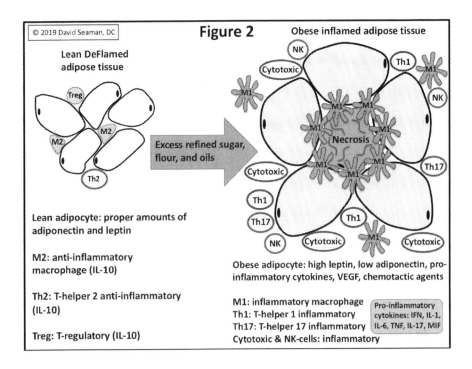

Elevated levels IL-17 promote multiple conditions, such as breast and other cancers, multiple sclerosis, rheumatoid arthritis, fatty liver, psoriasis, and autism.[16,17] Take note of the title of the following article published in the journal Science, which is one of the most respected of all journals.

> Estes ML, McAllister AK. Maternal Th17 cells take a
> toll on baby's brain. Science. 2016;351:919-20.

In this particular article, the authors describe how autoimmune and infection chemistry, which is identical to obesity chemistry, causes maternal Th17 immune cells to release IL-17 that bathe the baby's brain and can lead to autism.

In the next section of this chapter, we are going to look at the predisposing factors within the child that can promote autism. Exactly which factors are most important is not known at this point. However, we do know enough to outline preventive measures as well as what to focus on for autistic kids. In short, the preventive and so-called treatment approach would be the same; that is, to do everything possible to reduce the pro-inflammatory state.

The autism-prone developing child
While there are likely to be more predisposing factors than what I list below, these are the ones I have identified as participating in the expression of the autism, which are similar to those that cause breast cancer and other chronic diseases:

1. Autism genes[18-20]
2. Neuroinflammation[21-24]
3. Mitochondrial disorders[22,25-27]
4. Methylation issues[28,29]
5. Digestive inflammation[21,30,31]
6. Antioxidant imbalances[22,28,29,32]
7. Vitamin D deficiency[33,34]
8. Excess brain arachidonic acid[21,35,36]

Most of the predisposing factors listed above have been already discussed in this book in their respective chapters. My suggestion is to re-read those chapters by mentally replacing the term breast cancer with autism, and then you will have a good understanding for the causes of both breast cancer and autism.

Multiple studies have identified genes that make a child prone to autism.[18-20] I bring this up because it is important to understand that we are predisposed to various diseases based on our genetic makeup. This does not guarantee that we will get these diseases, but it does mean that we are more likely to express one or more of these diseases if we "flame up" beyond a tolerable level. As stated several times previously in this book, the way you identify if you are flaming is to track the well-known markers of inflammation that were detailed in *The DeFlame Diet* book.

Neuroinflammation in the child is based on the presence of autism genes, mitochondrial disorders (also genetically determined), methylation issues (also genetically determined) and maternal inflammation status. Only maternal inflammation is a modifiable risk factor and is the responsibility of the mother to address this issue before and during pregnancy. After the child is born, it can be further "flamed up" by a diet that creates digestive inflammation, antioxidant deficiencies, vitamin D deficiency, and an excess of omega-6 fatty acids. Sadly, these imbalances are created by the primary calories consumed by people age 2-years and older, which include desserts made with sugar and flour, bread, chicken, sugar sweetened beverages, pizza, and pasta.[37] A lack of anti-inflammatory vegetation and an excess of refined sugar, flour, and oils has been a consistent dietary trend for decades, which is why breast cancer, autism, depression, chronic pain, and all other chronic diseases continue to rise in prevalence.

If you want to do all you can to prevent autism or help a child with autism, all pro-inflammatory eating should be eliminated by the parents before conception, during the pregnancy, and thereafter for the parents and the new baby. Blaming vaccines and/or gluten as "the" cause(s) of autism is not a correct view to maintain.

Gluten and autism

I rarely eat gluten and the reason is because gluten grains (wheat, rye, and barley) and other whole grains provide the least amount of nutrients per calorie. It is much more nutritious to get our calories from vegetables, roots/tubers, fruit, meat, fish, chicken, nuts, and legumes. I describe this in detail in *The DeFlame Diet* book and also devoted a chapter to gluten, so I will not repeat the details herein.

The problem with gluten-free research for autism or any other condition is that researchers fail to capture an important issue – that is, they typically replace gluten with non-gluten flour or grain products. Anyone at any age with digestive inflammation, as described in Chapter 10 in this book and Chapter 15 in *The DeFlame Diet* book, typically does not respond well to starchy carbohydrate-rich whole grains and refined grains, as well as refined sugar and omega-6 oils. It is surprising that researchers do not comprehend this which can lead to no improvements if gluten is removed because the dietary approach still delivers unwanted refined carbohydrates and inflammatory oils to the young gut, which, as described below, can have the same effect as eating gluten.

With the above in mind, many studies report that there is no benefit for autistic kids if they go gluten-free and/or dairy-free.[38] Other studies report that there are varying degrees of benefit.[39] The DeFlame approach to gluten is not solely based on such studies, and here is why. Multiple human diseases are associated with chromosome 16, such as breast cancer and other cancers, most autoimmune diseases, and various diseases of the nervous system, such as Lou Gehrig's disease, multiple sclerosis, and autism.[40] A substance called zonulin localizes to chromosome 16, which is why zonulin production is considered to be a driver of most of the diseases associated with chromosome 16. In this 2010 study,[40] it was not clear if zonulin was associated with autism. In 2017, a study suggested that such a relationship exists.[41]

Gluten consumption is known to be one of the primary promoters of zonulin production,[40] which places those with celiac disease or gluten sensitivity at risk for developing chromosome 16-related diseases. The other primary driver of zonulin production is an excess of intestinal bacteria,[40] which is typically caused by overeating refined sugar, flour, and omega-6 oils. This is why I think it is wise to avoid gluten grains (wheat, rye, and barley) and non-gluten grains, and refined sugar, flour, and omega-6 oils. Part of *The DeFlame Diet* approach is to avoid zonulin production; there is no point in taking the risk. Life is too short as it is, and it makes no sense to adopt lifestyle choices that may promote additional pain, suffering, and misery.

Vaccines and autism
It is important to understand that vaccines are not required for autism to develop in a child. I have met several parents who did not vaccinate their kids and they still developed autism. For example, I met a father of 6-year old twin boys who explained to me that during his wife's pregnancy, she developed pneumonia and later a fairly intense urinary tract infection. The parents decided not to vaccinate their boys. Nonetheless, despite being vaccine-free, both boys developed autism, which speaks to the fact that blaming vaccines as "the" cause of autism is quite foolish. Both boys likely developed autism because they were unfortunately bathed in a pro-inflammatory infection environment for most of the pregnancy.

To the issue of whether or not vaccines can participate in the expression of autism, the answer is yes, and Drs. Sanjay Gupta and Jonathan Poling discussed this on CNN in 2008. You can watch the interview on YouTube by searching the internet for the following:

CNN's Dr. Sanjay Gupta interviews Dr. Jon Poling on 4-4-08

Dr. Poling's daughter, Hanna, immediately regressed into an autistic state after being vaccinated at 18 months of age. For this, the Poling family was compensated based on a determination by the vaccine court that was set up in the 1980's to pay for vaccine-related injuries.[42] At the time of the interview in 2008, there were nearly 5000 other autism claims pending in the court.[42] In Hanna's case, it was determined that she had a genetic mitochondrial disorder, which predisposed her to autism if her immune system was adequately activated. In her case, the nine routinely administered vaccines led to a robust enough immune response to cause Hanna to regress into an autistic state.[42] Subsequently, Dr. Poling and his colleagues wrote an article about mitochondrial disorders and autism expression.[25]

It does not appear anytime soon that the government will pull back on mandatory vaccine regulations, as most kids do not develop autism. My suggestion is that parents should fortify themselves and their children by being as DeFlamed as possible to reduce the likelihood of a child suffering an excessive immune response after being vaccinated, which could potentially push a child into an autistic state.

References
1. Franceschi C. Inflammaging as a major characteristic of old people: can it be prevented or cured? Nutr Rev. 2007 Dec;65(12 Pt 2):S173-6.
2. Franceschi C, Capri M, Monti D, et al. Inflammaging and anti-inflammaging: a systemic perspective on aging and longevity emerged from studies in humans. Mech Ageing Dev. 2007;128:92–105.
3. De Martinis M, Franceschi C et al. Inflamm-ageing and lifelong antigenic load as major determinants of ageing rate and longevity. FEBS Lett. 2005;579(10):2035-9.
4. Franceschi C, Bonafe MMecha, Valensin S et al. Inflamm-aging. An evolutionary perspective on immunosenescence. Ann N Y Acad Sci. 2000; 908:244-54.
5. Bjorklund G et al. Immune dysfunction and neuroinflammation in autism spectrum disorder. Acta Neurobiol Exp. 2016;76:257-68.
6. Goines P, Van de Water J. The immune system's role in the biology of autism. Curr Opin Neurol. 2010;23:111-17.
7. Scott O, Shi D, Andriashek D, Clark B, Goez HR. Clinical clues for autoimmunity and neuroinflammation in patients with autistic regression. Dev Med Child Neurol. 2017;59:947-51.
8. Gesundeheit B et al. Immunological and autoimmune considerations in autism spectrum disorders. J Autoimmunity. 2013;44:1-7.
9. Al-Ayadhi LY, Mostafa GA. Elevated serum levels of interleukin-17A in children with autism. J Neuroinflammation. 2012;9:158.
10. Xu N, Li X, Zhong Y. Inflammatory cytokines: potential biomarkers of immune dysfunction in autism spectrum disorders. Mediators Inflamm. 2015; Article ID 531518.

11. Keil A et al. Parental autoimmune diseases associated with autism spectrum disorders in offspring. Epidemiology. 2010;21:805-808.

12. Cutolo M. Sex hormone adjuvant therapy in rheumatoid arthritis. Rheum Dis Clin North Am. 2000;26:881-95.

13. van der Burg JW et al. The role of systemic inflammation linking maternal body mass index to neurodevelopment in children: inflammation and neurodevelopment. Pediatr Res. 2016;79:3-12.

14. Li M, Fallin MD, Riley A, et al. The association of maternal obesity and diabetes with autism and other developmental disabilities. Pediatrics. 2016;137(2):e20152206.

15. Sanchez CD, Barry C, Sabhlok A, et al. Maternal pre-pregnancy obesity and child neurodevelopmental outcomes: a meta-analysis. Obes Rev. 2018;19:464-84.

16. Chehimi M, Vidal H, Eljaafari A. Pathogenic role of IL-17-producing immune cells in obesity, and related inflammatory diseases. J Clin Med. 2017;6(7). pii: E68.

17. Estes ML, McAllister AK. Maternal Th17 cells take a toll on baby's brain. Science. 2016;351:919-20.

18. Gupta S, Ellis Se, Ashar FN, et al. Transcriptome analysis reveals dysregulation of innate immune response genes and neuronal activity-dependent genes in autism.

19. de la Torre-Ubieta L, Won H, Stein JL, et al. Advancing the understanding of autism disease mechanisms through genetics. Nat Med. 2016;22:345-61.

20. Voineagu I, Wang X, Johnston P, et al. Transcriptomic analysis of autistic brain reveals convergent molecular pathology. Nature. 2013;474:380-84.

21. Madore C et al. Neuroinflammation in autism: plausible role of maternal inflammation, dietary omega 3, and microbiota. Neural Plasticity. 2016; Article ID: 3597209.

22. Rossignol DA, Frye RE. A review of research trends in physiological abnormalities in autism spectrum disorders: immune dysregulation, inflammation, oxidative stress, mitochondrial dysfunction and environmental toxicant exposures. Mol Psychiatry. 2012;17(4):389-401.

23. Young AM, et al. Aberrant NF-kappaB expression in autism spectrum condition: a mechanism for neuroinflammation. Frontiers Psychiatry. 2011; May 13;2:27

24. Young AM et al. From molecules to neural morphology: understanding neuroinflammation in autism spectrum condition. Mol Autism. 2016; Jan 20;7:9.

25. Poling JS, Frye RE, Shoffner J, Zimmerman AW. Developmental regression and mitochondrial dysfunction in a child with autism. J Child Neurol. 2006;21(2):170-72.

26. Weissman JR, Kelley RI, Bauman ML et al. Mitochondrial disease in autism spectrum disorder patients: a cohort analysis. PLoS ONE. 2008;3(11):e3815

27. Swaminathan N. Vaccine injury case offers a clue to the cause of autism. Sci Am. April 22, 2008. https://www.scientificamerican.com/article/vaccine-injury-case-offer/

28. Rose S, et al. Intracellular and extracellular redox status and free radical generation in primary immune cells from children with autism. Autism Res Treat. 2012;2012:986519.

29. James SJ, et al. Metabolic biomarkers of increased oxidative stress and impaired methylation capacity in children with autism. Am J Clin Nutr. 2004;80:1611-7.

30. Luna RA et al. Distinct microbiome-neuroimmune signatures correlate with functional abdominal pain in children with autism spectrum disorder. Cell Mol Gastroenterol Hepatol. 2016;3(2):218-230.

31. Frye RE, et al. Gastrointestinal dysfunction in autism spectrum disorder: the role of mitochondria and the enteric microbiome. Microbial Ecol Health Dis. 2016;26:27458.

32. Frye RE, James SJ. Metabolic pathology of autism in relation to redox metabolism. Biomarkers Med. 2014;8:321-30.

33. Vinkhuyzen AA et al. Gestational vitamin D deficiency and autism spectrum disorder. BJPsych OPEN. 2017;3:85-90.

34. Saad K et al. Vitamin D status in autism spectrum disorders and the efficacy of vitamin D supplementation in autistic children. Nutr Neurosci. 2016;19:346-51.

35. Tamiji J, Crawford DA. The neurobiology of lipid metabolism in autism spectrum disorders. Neurosignals. 2010;18:98-112.

36. Parletta N, Niyonsenga T, Duff J. Omega-3 and omega-6 polyunsaturated gatty acid levels and correlations with symptoms in children with attention deficit hyperactivity disorder, autistic spectrum disorder and typically developing controls. PLoS One. 2016;11(5):e0156432.

37. US Department of Agriculture, US Department of Health and Human Services. Dietary Guidelines for Americans 2010.

38. Elder JH, Kreider CM, Schaefer NM, de Laosa MB. A review of gluten- and casein-free diets for treatment of autism: 2005-2015. Nutr Diet Suppl. 2015;7:87-101.

39. Whiteley P, Shattock P, Knivsberg AM, et al. Gluten- and casein-free dietary intervention for autism spectrum conditions. Front Hum Neurosci. 2013;6:344.

40. Fasano A. Zonulin and its regulation of intestinal barrier function: the biological door to inflammation, autoimmunity, and cancer. Physiol Rev. 2011;91:151-75.

41. Esnafoglu E, Cirrik S, Ayyildiz SN, et al. Increased serum zonulin levels as an intestinal permeability marker in autistic subjects. J Pediatr. 2017;188:240-44.

42. CNN. Vaccine case draws new attention to autism debate. March 7, 2008. http://www.cnn.com/2008/HEALTH/conditions/03/06/vaccines.autism/index.html

Chapter 18
Putting it all together

After reading the previous 17 chapters, my hope is that you have come to the logical conclusion that many factors are involved in creating the pro-inflammatory state that promotes breast cancer. You should now realize how multiple pro-inflammatory lifestyle choices can coalesce to create a tidal wave of inflammation that pushes breast cancer to emerge.

On a personal note, as stated in the introduction, in 2009 my mother dealt with a grade 1 ductal carcinoma in situ, which means it was localized without any evidence of spreading to the lymphatic system or anywhere else. She went through radiation treatments and since then, there has been no evidence of reemergence locally or elsewhere; so, our family was lucky. She read this book before we went to print and she had no idea that so many pro-inflammatory factors were involved in breast cancer expression, and more importantly, her personal physician and oncologist never told her about any of the information in this book, or *The DeFlame Diet* or in *Weight Loss Secrets You Need To Know*.

My mother had previously read *The DeFlame Diet*; however, the information in that book did not specifically register in her mind as being directly related to breast cancer, which is why I wrote this book...for her and all women who go through life without this important information, only to be blind-sided by the diagnosis of breast cancer after years of engaging in lifestyle choices that are overtly pro-inflammatory and pro-cancerous, but take time to finally emerge as a potentially catastrophic and life-threatening disease.

The DeFlame Diet for Breast Health and Cancer Prevention is the first of my condition-specific *DeFlame* books. Each will be about 100 pages long, which means they are of a moderate length because they focus specifically on the important inflammatory details related to a specific condition. If I were to include in this book all of the action steps for DeFlaming, as outlined in *The DeFlame Diet* book and in the *Weight Loss Secrets* book, this breast health book would be over 450 pages long.

My next book will be about depression, which is also a chronic pro-inflammatory state, and will also be about 100 pages long. If I was to include in the depression book all of the action steps for DeFlaming, as outlined in *The DeFlame Diet* and in *Weight Loss Secrets*, the book about depression would also be over 450 pages long.

In short, the human mind learns better if we upload information in learnable chunks that are related to each other, so as to build a solid foundation of knowledge upon which we can build. *The DeFlame Diet* book is specifically about how food increases or decreases inflammation and provides guidelines for achieving and maintaining a DeFlamed state, no matter what condition you may be suffering from or are trying to prevent from emerging.

Not everyone is overweight or obese, so it would have been foolish to have 100 pages of information about weight loss secrets in *The DeFlame Diet*. The *Weight Loss Secrets* book is actually about arming our brains with information so that a state of mindfulness can dominate the eating domain of our lives. To achieve and maintain a DeFlamed body weight, you need to specifically understand the obesogenic environment and the constant eating stimuli to which we are all exposed, which come in the form of advertisements, inflammatory drives, emotional drives, and primordial drives. Without combating the various weight-gain stimuli, it is very difficult to maintain a DeFlamed body weight.

So, clearly, the reason why you chose to read this present book is because you are concerned about breast health. Now that you know the details about why/how breast cancer is a pro-inflammatory state, you need to read *The DeFlame Diet* book and do everything you can to achieve a DeFlamed state. Whether or not you need to read *Weight Loss Secrets You Need To Know* depends on whether or not you are overweight or obese. If you do not have a weight problem, there is little need to read *Weight Loss Secrets*, except for the fact that it is very interesting, with information you may not be aware of regarding how and why most eat in the fashion they do, and to help you prevent an overweight/obese state in your lifetime, or that of a loved one.

You should have noticed that there was virtually no information in this breast health book about nutritional supplements. The reason is because there are no specific supplements that exclusively target breast tissue. Supplements should be taken with the mindset of inflammation reduction, which is briefly discussed in the next chapter.

Chapter 19
Anti-inflammatory supplements

People tend to have misperceptions about nutritional supplements, which likely exist due to how we perceive how medications work. We have been conditioned to perceive that drugs are taken to treat the name of a disease. This is actually quite inaccurate. Drugs either augment or inhibit biochemical pathways associated with a given disease. The difference is not a trivial semantic issue. I say this because people routinely look for supplements to treat their diseases instead of taking medications. The missing piece in this thought process is a lack of knowledge about the inflammatory state of the individual with the disease.

Long before a specific disease manifests, people live in a chronic inflammatory state as outlined in this book, and in even greater detail in *The Deflame Diet* book. Drugs essentially target the abnormal metabolism of a given organ or system after it manifests due to chronic inflammation. In other words, the underlying chronic inflammation, which is the cause of the disease, is not typically addressed. For example, in the case of breast cancer, women are treated with drugs that have estrogen-inhibiting mechanisms, such as aromatase inhibitors (Arimidex, Aromasin, Femara) or estrogen receptor blockers (Tamoxifen, Fareston). These drugs do not address the underlying chronic inflammatory state that promoted the pro-inflammatory changes that occur in estrogen metabolism.

The DeFlame approach is to essentially ignore the name of the disease and focus on reducing inflammation to normal. This means that we should also essentially ignore the name of a disease when taking supplements to reduce inflammation. With this in mind, some of the key supplements to reduce inflammation have already been discussed, including iodine (Chapter 12), vitamin D (Chapter 13), and omega-3 fatty acids from fish oil (Chapter 15). I take all of the supplements discussed in this chapter for the precise purpose of inflammation reduction.

Probiotics (Lactobacillus and Bifidobacteria) were briefly mentioned in Chapter 10. To date the exact formula and supplemental dose to get the best DeFlaming effect is not known. My perception is that we should focus on the readily available probiotics, the most notable being Lactobacillus acidophilus and Bifidobacterium.

Studies continue to emerge that highlights how low magnesium intake is associated with inflammation.[1-3] The precise amount that we should supplement with is not known. The general range is 400-1000 mg per day. Whether or not someone with cancer should take magnesium is debatable. While it appears that adequate magnesium intake appears to help prevent many inflammatory conditions, such as diabetes, heart disease, and cancer, it also appears that established tumors can be stimulated by magnesium.[4] Consider that cancer cells tend to have high concentrations of magnesium, which is needed for glycolysis (Chapter 5) and other metabolic pathways.[4] So, if I had cancer, I am not sure if I would take magnesium. I think scientists should investigate magnesium supplementation in animal models of cancer that compared a ketogenic and non-ketogenic diet. This would help determine the viability of supplementing with magnesium if one had cancer.

Coenzyme Q10 (CoQ10) has anti-inflammatory and antioxidant functions.[5] CoQ10 also helps mitochondria create energy (ATP) and has an anti-aging effect on skeletal muscle.[6] The typical supplemental recommendation is 100 mg per day.

Anti-inflammatory botanicals, such as ginger and turmeric, have been known for a long time to exert anti-inflammatory effects. This has generally become common knowledge. The typical recommendation is 1 or more grams per day of individual or combination of products.

As stated above, I take all of these supplements for the purpose of supporting my DeFlame Diet. I do not take them for any particular symptom or condition, but instead, solely for the purpose of their anti-inflammatory effects.

References

1. Sugimoto J, Romani AM, Valentin-Torres AM, et al. Magnesium decreases inflammatory cytokine production: a novel innate immunomodulatory mechanism. J Immunol. 2012;188:6338-46.
2. Weglicki WB. Hypomagnesemia and inflammation: clinical and basic aspects. Ann Rev Nutr. 2012;32:55–71.
3. Nielson FH. Magnesium deficiency and increased inflammation: current perspectives. J Inflamm Res. 2018;11:25-34.
4. Castiglioni S, Maier JA. Magnesium and cancer: a dangerous liason. Mag Res. 2011;24:S92-S100.
5. Zhai J, Bo Y, Lu YU, Liu C, Zhang L. Effects of coenzyme Q10 on markers of inflammation: a systemic review and meta-analysis. PLoS One. 2017;12:e0170172.
6. Linnane AW, Zhang C, Yarovaya N, et al. Human aging and global function of coenzyme Q10. Ann NY Acad Sci. 2002;959:396-411.

Chapter 20
Sobering facts about breast cancer and disease in general

Because we use the term "healthcare system," we mistakenly believe that we have a health promotion system...we don't. Our medical system is here to support us after we "pursue and achieve" cancer and other chronic diseases. In the case of my mother's breast cancer, several of us went to the treatment planning session with the oncologist. The doctor only discussed the therapeutic intervention with radiation and NOTHING else. Nothing about what to eat or not to eat – absolutely NOTHING. And there is a reason for this; our healthcare system is actually a disease-care system. In my opinion, this is absolutely fine as long as you know this is the case and you also know that your family's healthcare is on you and no one else.

If you choose to pursue disease and you achieve that goal, you have a disease-care system waiting for you to give money to. If you properly pursue health, then you can mostly avoid the disease-care system for the majority of your life, which will save you thousands of dollars and the associated pain and suffering related to the disease and its treatment.

In the United States, disease-care, which is euphemistically called healthcare, is a $3.5 trillion-dollar industry. Multiple billions are spent on breast health and breast cancer. The scientific search for breast cancer and other disease cures is specifically directed at creating new and expensive medications. This ideology exists because the disease-care system centers around people making really bad lifestyle choices, which eventually causes people to need expensive medications and treatments.

It is foolish for people to wait around for magical cures to appear from the disease-care industry because this is not the purpose of the industry. You have to realize that we have a "disease-care" system...not a health promotion system. In other words, your health is on you – it is your choice to pursue disease or to pursue health. If you want to avoid breast cancer, then you need to get as DeFlamed as possible, which is not a 100% guarantee; it just greatly increases your odds of not developing breast cancer or any other chronic disease.

When it comes to patients who see a doctor, 60% or more are typically women. Guys typically avoid going to the doctor at all costs. It is not uncommon for a doctor to ask a new male patient why he is here today, and the man says, "because my wife made me." With this in mind, women who want to avoid or better manage breast cancer, you have the power to change the inflammatory status of your kitchen. You can DeFlame it. If you do this, you will help your husband avoid diseases like prostate cancer, since it too is driven by chronic inflammation.

If you have kids, DeFlaming your kitchen will prevent acne expression in your children, which can be particularly traumatic for teens. If you have children who are athletic, *The DeFlame Diet* is ideal because the outcome of aggressive training and athletic events is low-grade tissue trauma, which requires repair. The body's repair process is all about controlling inflammation.

In short, if you DeFlame your diet, you will give yourself and family the best chance of avoiding pain, depression, and chronic disease. You will create an anti-inflammatory buffer to protect your family from the ravages of the disease itself and the over-priced treatments you will otherwise have to endure. My suggestion is to essentially memorize, or at least become very familiar, with the information in this book, *The DeFlame Diet*, and *Weight Loss Secrets You Need To Know*.

Index